Bedtime St

Stressed Out Adults

Relaxing Sleep Stories for Anxiety Relief, Deep Sleep Hypnosis. Guided Mindfulness Meditation to Help Adults Falling Asleep Fast with Self-Healing Techniques

Winifred Campbell

Table of Contents

The Canal of Utrecht

We will wander through the historic Dutch city of Utrecht. It is a city of cobblestones and culture that, like always, they can pleasantly and conveniently close their eyes first, relax their arms, legs, fingers, and toes. Feel how the muscles have released the already tense residues from the day allows your bones to fall? When you inhale deeply and exhale at your own pace. You can imagine every thought as if a cloud floating in the sky above it will come and go. You can watch if he will pass by the time he leaves, another will replace him, then you will separate from these clouds. There will be some distance between you and your thoughts. With bright golden edges, rays of light come out from all sides, feeling how the light falls on your face, it bends you here. Where you are swooning. You feel a hard surface. Severely you look down to find an old stone bridge over the sky near soft blue and gold decorated with small puffy clouds—a beautiful day in the Dutch city of Utrecht. The bridge crosses one of the canals of the city that surrounds the city center to your left - a small row of shops made of white stone.

Your right brick rows of houses are aligned along the edge of the canal. The sky is big and full of movement. The wind catches the clouds and pushes them through the blue background every few minutes when one of the large clouds whips in front of the sun. How old you look up and see how the edge of one such darkness turns from grey to gold? When the sun illuminates it from behind the veil, casts a shadow on the ground. You feel how your cheeks turn from warm to cool. You close your eyes, and light plays on your eyelids. When the clouds move away from the sun. The temperature rises so much that it warms the tip of the nose. When you get used to the fact that the clouds move again, even when your eyes are closed, you can follow the dynamic movements of the sky from the shadow warm to cool, when the dust passes through the corner of the sky. The light on the back eyelids darkens slightly on the right. The breeze slightly touches your hair. You open your eyes from the bridge stretching out in a confusing city, laid in front of you. Now you understand where artists of the Dutch golden age drew inspiration.

 The quality of light is unusual. You can imagine the same sky stretched over a wheat field with one tree. It's possible by playing a game of light and shadow in a small village with hay bales stacked at a bar in the distance, and possibly clouds tracing their way through a brick in a stone city. Such as this one, with shops and houses, canals, and Spiers of beautiful churches the dashed horizon, as soon as this thought comes to your mind. In the bowels of the cathedral chimes nearby the sounds along the winding calling stone roads of the city. The echoes of high and low notes are intertwined with a hail of intestines from the tower, above which it stands above the shops. Your right too, In fact, it is the tallest building in all of Utrecht, which for centuries has been the unwritten rule in the city. Nothing is higher than the bell tower of this mighty cathedral. It is the central part of the horizon. Here it rises a hundred meters in height. As the highest view in all the Netherlands, it was built in thirteen hundred as the crown. Many people now call Martin's Cathedral his home church. Still, this tower is separate from the rest of the cathedral, and behind it is a detached nave. Martin's cathedral collapsed in sixteen hundred, leaving the tower separated from the main building. Therefore, it stands tall, square, and lonely since the two lower parts of the tower are rectangular. The third and highest part is Lacy.

Open the frieze here, sending the sounds of bells all over Utrecht. They can be heard nearby where you are standing. On the outskirts of the city gives way to fields and a farm you exit the bridge and follow the bells to the church from the cobblestone streams flow from the canal. You will not slowly enjoy the unique sound of steps on the stone, strengths, and small things, as well as clothes decorated with fancy shops. There are a coffee shop and a short saying made of lace and fabric—a chocolate shop filled with beautiful cakes and pies on a full glass window. People sit at small tables at the sun of the cafe, lazily leaf through the morning newspaper. Others talk with friends, quietly laugh at a personal joke, smile when you go, this is a lively city, friendly. They are hospitable. Maybe it would be nice to stay in one of the cafes, which, in your opinion. The Bastille did not take well after you explore a little more of the city, the path of which runs under the arch under it. The Dog Tower, on the other hand, opens to the charming square town along which there are cafes and shops.

This is the place where Nayar used to be. The space between the two parts of the church turns into a cozy gathering place in beautiful weather. Today from here, you are walking along a road that gently descends to the left, as it will not let you down; the lobby paves cobblestones under your feet. Cyclists pass some generals leading their friends into the street to warn you that there are so many. Bicycles here, in fact, some say that there are more bicycles than people. The Netherlands is a small country and very flat, so cycling makes sense. What freedom do you think to ride a bicycle and go exploring before the street takes you to the exit, which is the old canal? This is the heart of the city in the mornings of the weekend. The streets on both sides of the old canal turn into an open market. Where you can find people who sang apple pies, covered with small puff donors, powdered sugar, and a stream, on each corner are hundreds of stalls with large metal buckets tucked with tulips.

Yellow, why are pink and purple tulips that you can wrap in paper to take home and put Avars on your kitchen table on market days. When people are busy, but here in the early evening, a quiet old canal in Utrecht is different from many canals that you will find in the big cities of the Netherlands. Not only has roads that follow it higher, but there is also a path on both sides to the Black metal staircase of the water level leading from the streets to the water edge.

You choose one such sadist, as he hears, as iron metal bounces with every step, and below, you see large black wooden double doors on either side of the water. These were old warehouses for storing hoops delivered by boat to the city. You imagine what could have been stormed outside these doors, and days, spices, tea, root crops, and grains have passed. Now these old ones under Army I have turned into faint music notes of live music coming from one of the satyrs behind you into restaurants and cafes. I had a traditional Dutch pancake restaurant, a kitchen, the main dining room in response a lunch peak is already on the way. Hence, the waiters set up a table, chairs, and the edge of the canal through which you go to the restaurant and look at the menu. Dutch pancakes are similar to giant crabs. They can be obtained with an assortment of savory and sweet fillings, such as apple and cheese mushrooms, pineapple, and one with a variety of herbs, like chocolate for dessert or berries and cream. You also get a traditional pancake with rich dark syrup. You will always find Aaron at all. You know, the bottle sounds as if you are not mistaken here, you take. Sitting at one of the tables closest to the waiter, the waiter comes with a pleasant smile and accepts your order. You pick one of the pancakes that looked especially good on the menu and picked a good cold drink through the canal.

Like a family of ducks sitting on a brick ledge near the water, one disheveled, like feathers and other suitors, the third just decided to go for a swim. If he flies his wings slightly and lands on the surface of the canal with a smooth movement. The ripples in the pastries lazily wake up legs of me. As she slowly crosses the canal in search of a snack. She crawls past a handful of leaves that have fallen into the water. The leaves have sharp edges. You can rotate them, like a stream gently throwing them from side to side. They look like small rafts for dragonflies descending along a mighty river. But if the leaves were broken, the ducks would be the size of a duelist, Uncas, how funny the world looks when you see it from a different angle. You are not sure how long you watch the family of ducks doing their evening things. You pay attention to time, but after a while, the waiter returns with food. The pancake arrives on a huge boom and white ceramic dish, while the pancakes are thin and tender.

They are quite big ones. In size, it looks just amazing; you enjoy the first bite. The combination of tastes does not look like what you tried before. It's just beautiful that the food warms you as the evening air starts to cool when you finish dinner. You look through Channel one small Ducks are now all in the water, following the current. When he takes them from under a small stone bridge, you wave to them when they pass. One of them turns to you in the crack, you imagine it and, perhaps, wish you good in the evening. Which makes you smile, now it's time to go your way to thank the waiter for the food and climb the stairs to the main street, for a little darker. The street of lies starts to flicker one by one along with the canal, and down to the cobbled streets, there is a store. In which a rental-purchase has just left you, and after lunch, moving sounds more than sparkling. He chooses a bicycle that has the correct height and which blocks the wheel with a small key. Which makes a soft one by clicking on it, jump on it and easily adjust it seat, pushing it forward, and starting the pedal from the old channel. This city is primarily flat and teeming with bicycle paths that provide smooth riding. You enjoy using your hands and feet, and Suddenly your breeze blows past your hair when it turns left and right. You pedal again under straight eyes and walk past rows of trees.

Where the birds camp, waiting for a snack. He has paths and classic Dutch houses with fancy intricate tongs on the roofs in the summer around. Some have small arches in their tongues. They remind you of the top hats on wedding cakes, how they stand out - Dwight - and red buildings. He walked past the statue of a rabbit and the State Theater and spoke on the road leading to Rye past grocery stores and shopping centers through which you cross smaller canals and small parks that cross between residential streets. After one crossing, you get to a much larger enclosure, so named Wilhelminsky park for the famous Dutch king, you are here. In the center of a lush green lawn, her famous statue stands. She is wrapped in a coat and hat. She looks quite regal when the black road passes by you. You go to the next part of the city. This is a residential area with small quiet streets dotted within individual houses. The full windows of each house radiate a warm glow through the open curtains to the road inside the table, where they are sold for dinner—the rows of bookshelves on the walls of the living room.

A bridge with unusual decorations, the front side of which is laid from top to bottom with square white tiles, each of which has its luger. There is so much art, and often in the most unexpected As long as this is your favorite part of the city. It seems to you that you continue to grow past the bushes with pink and purple flowers past the entire brick wall. Where the shiny iron gates leading to the campus. You see students sitting outside on the lawn watching the day turn into night and soft blankets in the summer, reading what surrounds talking with friends or playing card games. You turned right and walked along the bike path away from the main road leading to a forest path by a long lazy river. The river is narrow as a canal. The stream rises, green to

—

your left, water flows along the coast, sometimes whitening. Where it passes along the roots of tango trees, hangs over a bench.

The air is fresh and clean. Here you can smell the moist earth and wet leaves mixed with the fragrant aroma of flowers. The path leads you deeper into the forest, small lights and soil lead you to hear the sounds of birth, reconciled for the night and a small animal. Returning to his burrows in front, he sees warm light through the trees. What can be surprising when you are approaching. You understand that the city, located in the center of the forest, asked everyone the glass walls. The fireplace in the corner that people spoke about cozy tables, warming your hands-on hot teacups, with a colorfully painted tea box hanging on hooks by the fire. You park your bike at the return desk near the entrance, and, going into the tears inside, utter calm chatter and clinking ceramic cups that you order pots with your favorite type of tea and take it out on a tray. The lawn of the tea house gently descends to the river bank, which you followed here. You sent one of the tables next to small water boats in any direction there are groups of friends, families and individual travelers who spend a pleasant evening for a relaxing paddle up and down the river as soon as the tea has cooled a little. You pour yourself a cup and enjoy the feeling when your hands on the outside of the mug fill the uterus from the inside. When you take the set, everyone sees you and also from the inside.

The smell of tea rises to your nose a steaming from a pot that you think is very cold. You saw today a dawn tower, shops, and intricate gable houses, duck families for an evening swim. You smile, thinking about them. You remember the delicious pancake that I still feel how pleasant aromas are at the tip of your tongue after you have finished drinking tea. You heard it from the riverbank. You listen to the sound of the flowing river and the small ripples in the water's edge attention. He offers us to ride a boat up and down the rivers and canals of Utrecht, you ask about returning to the city in this way and tells you, of course, yes the guide and binds the green. The child's boat and puts plush white pillows on the wooden seats. He enters the boat and sits, feeling immersed in the softness of the cushion beneath you. When the guide comes and lifts the wooden oars on both sides of the guide. You walk along the lazy river past the tea house and return to the forest. The river spins and turns left or right among the trees, while you listen to the sound of rowing behind you. Something pleasant in a soft rhythmic whirlpool throughout the water. You think that it will take you some time to return to the city.

The guide says you, and many people use the ride to take a nap. You feel a little sleepy. You think it was all day to explore this beautiful city. The boat gently sways back and forth in the rhythm of an oar pulling beneath the surface of the water, which is landing quietly on the sides of the ship. You feel the eyelids become heavy, you slide further into the pillows and allow yourself to relax. You feel safe and comfortable. Now it's dark, and the ladder has appeared above your head. You lean back to look at this black canvas from above, but before the lamb changes into the darkness behind your tired eyelids, Utrecht's beauty and the boats rocking back and forth, like in a cradle for safe and calm sleep.

Treehouse by The Ocean

When you find yourself in Madagascar, you can surrender and restore communication with nature and with yourself in the safety of an ancient dwelling on bail of the Bob tree—uniting the miracle of life in the hollow of an old and respected tree. You can calmly fall asleep over the Indian Ocean and under the majestic African sky. A person binds the reins and allows your imagination to fly up. You can remember that you forgot that you control your thoughts, and they communicate your feelings. So let's take a look at the beauty of imagination before sailing across the bridge from your awakening life to your dreams, and drowsiness becomes more comfortable in your bed, feeling it's hard when you go down. You can take any lasting impression of your day, close your eyes and let your eyelids feel like cold heavy sandbags. Your tired eyes present your whole body soothingly from head to toe a feeling of relaxation. You can visualize the linen-covered storage box in your favorite pattern and color scheme. You can take the deepest breath of the day and then blow the air through your lips. As if blowing through the straw directly into this box. You can see your breathing like a hot stream on which all your thoughts, problems, and anxieties fall into a safe box again. Inhale and possibly yawn, letting your stomach rise eat before you blow out everything that you keep in your body filling this box. You can take a soft one if it is lit and put it on top of the box.

All your worries and things that cannot be solved right now can be stored in this box. When you visualize its placement on a high shelf, or it can remain until the right time because the present moment is just for you to bask and relax when we go on vacation or mind. You can now imagine yourself covered with beams of deep honey tangerine sunlight that warms your face and illuminates the strands of your hair. As if they were immersed in gold, a light breeze, and dry. Thin blades feathered grass dark from above and green below tickle bare feet. Which are decorated with sandals in the distance? When you hear the ocean's rolling waves, like Hey, shatter on the shore, protecting your eyes from the late afternoon. The sun with your hand, you see the blue waters of the Indian Ocean in the distance. Some smells hate your nose. A sweet earth note can recognize them. They are new to you and unique. Only in Madagascar is the island of Madagascar, located off the coast of East Africa, located in the Indian Ocean. More than ninety percent of its wildlife is not found anywhere in the world, and this leads to a feeling of discovery, as you find yourself among tall bale of bean trees.

This line runs along a dirt road leading to your places of residence. These trees are ancient, some of them are very old. Their trunks are thick enough to serve as houses that go high into the sky, in front of the broad branches of lush green leaves, like clouds of foliage against the background of a deep forest. Blue skies in arid climates such as Madagascar, chests store water, while the very peaks are ideal for nesting the myth Around Veo Bob. A tree that was taken from the ground and then transplanted upside down. So that the roots that stretch to the sky over the bark, have healing properties in diseases of the stomach. Its leaves and fruits are considered the treatment of almost any condition. It is not surprising that this tree is referred to as the tree of life. Maybe Beans are sacred and revered that you follow a path that brings you closer to the ocean when the sun sets, and local birds sing in songs, praising another day. You experience the same feeling of gratitude and lightness as the heat of the day begins to come. You turn along the path that goes to the guarded residence. You stopped moving away from the rustic walk, carefully avoiding splitting the forest and finding a way surrounded by a garden where there are orchids and shades of fuchsia and Darwin's. Famous White Orchid seems almost like a flower from another planet with sharp dots that form a star and a central petal that looks like a falling white veil.

The air is filled with mixed perfumes of these exotic flowers that remind you of cooked raspberries, coconut, and sour green apples. You reach out and touch the thin and tiny petals of Madagascar's periwinkles, that feel small pieces of silk and hot pink in pastel purple-blue. You don't smile sweetly when your lips are relaxed and spontaneously bent up to the deep fiery-orange ball of the sun, which begins to set. You cannot believe in the magic of this late day since all this seems so new and yet, at the same time, closely connected with you. How amazing you felt? When the child looked like a fluffy subnet bumblebee from a flower. You continued to walk past the garden to see the ring-tailed lemur and running a child throughout the property. She stops curiously to meet your gaze. Although you are both warm with each other. There is mutual respect, her eyes, like large copper coins, are made romantic thanks to marks similar to a thick black eyeliner.

Her little faces turned red with white and grey spots on her tail puffs with excitement from smoke and ring charcoal. When our tiny child clings tightly to her back, people come from all over the world chance to meet local lemurs face to face. You are surprised that you have such a chance to hear her gently. It is felt before it rushes through a property radiated by sunlight. The sky is now covered with purple brushstrokes and Mellon and lavender as the day draws to a close. You continue along a narrow path that leads to a hill overlooking the Indian Ocean's aquamarine waters, and at the top of this hill is the Bayo Bob tree. Which was turned into a treehouse that challenges even the most imaginary of your childhood visions? This is a creation that combines the best nature design with the skill of the locals, created in the form of a silhouette against the background, the setting sun over the ocean. Which he reaches, letting through the saturated red, pink, and orange colors of the sky.

As if tall - a high-rise building, seeming taller than any tree you come across, standing alone and alone, and not in the forest, at the bottom of the pipe. It was partially hollowed out with an entrance that was carved in the shape of an arc that Bob could survive and live despite this since the thick bark and layers of cambium remain decades ago, the tree was saved from decay. The core and sculpted in the treehouse that stands today. The house has many levels without its decks, connected with spiral staircases with polished handrails of driftwood. From these decks, single vibrations hung a thick braided rope and mesh fabric of a hammock, hand-painted in shades of indigo. You go to the swing and a small mosaic table in cool blue and aquamarine tones. When the legs made of twisted, you go to the rhythm and a small mosaic tabletop in cool blue and aquamarine tones. Its legs are made of bentwood on the table - a cold glass bottle covered with condensation when drops water flows down it.

A drink is a sweet drink, next to it is a note from the owner, written on a form with an inscription that shows a sketch of a treehouse. Your name is elegantly written, as well as a message that we are delighted to receive if you enjoy the magic. At night you take a bottle, and you go to the hammock-swing, allowing you to weave the net around you in the desired embrace. Your body feels tired and sore tender, which pleases you, as a reminder of great adventures in the hot sun. This led you to this delay at the end of the day.

The rays of the ocean are soft and fresh. You like salt when a gentle fog hits your face when you plunge into a swing and surrender. The sun is

---

14

approaching the exit point, meeting a calm ocean and a haze of plums that form along the horizon. You bring the ice-cold glass bottle to your lips, feeling the drops of condensation that you like before sipping a sweet drink that drains into your throat and cools you as you want. A gentle waterfall suddenly discovered in the depths of humid tropical forest, you sway back and forth, bending, sighing, and letting go. The sky begins to darken. The moon starts to glow like a perfect whirlwind of buttercream falling on a lush and velvety black plum sky. Stars blaze sparkling because they shine brighter than you ever remember when fireflies rise in the air. In the glow of your tired, happy eyes, it seems like a rain of gold and silver shines pouring on you. At the same time, you continue to rock. You allow yourself to immerse yourself in a fabulous state with such a relaxed and educated vision that it is challenging to distinguish turns around you and rises above your head so that for a moment, you feel that you are flying in space. You take another sip from the bottle when the glass gently bangs on your teeth and pulls you out of the Madagascar spell. When you rise and let your feet balance on solid ground, ready to enter the treehouse for the night. The nap is that the bottle increases to the table and goes to the arch of the treehouse, which is now lit by chains of solar-powered lights that wrap around the deck above the head and flow from the railing in the form of loose strands, like lit willows of a weeping willow.

You watch the lights flow in the ocean before entering the hollow trunk of the tree inside the tree. The air is a little dry. You smell the sweet tree on the ground floor of the house is a kitchen with a modest pit in the center full of fuel; the walls of the tree are decorated. It is decorated with paintings of Madagascar, which depict images of tropical forests and open fields and scenes from the ocean. A tap was found in the wall from which water flows from inside the tree. You touch the tree around it, feeling that it is soft and moist. While other parts of the tree are stable and smooth. The collection of shells is in a bowl on the mosaic counter, which matches the ocean table outside. You go up to it and drag your fingers along the pattern, vibrant blue and green remind you of the mermaid tail—the colors of Indian oceans, which are continually changing throughout the day.

When you touch the seashells, enjoying the feeling of their crests and patterns. When they feel fresh in your hands, and next to the bowl of shells, there is a basket of sweet delicacies that smell like Madagascar vanilla, as well as a few pieces of baobab fruit. The fruit is as healthy as coconut. You open it, and the white chalk pods inside are dry, but it tastes pretty sweet. You feel tired and welcome a light snack that allows it to get enough. When you do not drink, you close your eyes and enjoy the security of this tree. Which more than the bedroom in which you were a small child, leaves you feeling surprised. The pleasure and pleasure of staying in this magical tree that has survived for centuries and still stands strong and resilient. As if it is empty, conveys all the energy and history of those who came before you flourished, and left their mark in history. Now this value, ancient Bob, witnessed all of this. He stood here alone, strong and independent. It makes you feel your own ability to climb, to be proud and healthy on your own. You feel respect and gratitude when you reach for a wooden staircase that rises the inside of the tree and leads you to the second floor. Your strong hands grab every step when you climb higher and higher sounds of the ocean, insects, and frogs. I will marry a night orchestra, which increases in volume.

When you arrive in the open-air living on the second floor, dimly lit by sparkling strings of lights, fireflies and stars are like the continuation of these tiny luminous balls. As again, you feel as if you are traveling to another galaxy. You go to the deck with an ocean view to find an open-air shower with a rain shower. There is a small rustic baby, on which fresh towels and a linen bathrobe are neatly folded. Next to shower is a handmade basket of handmade soap made from shea butter, cut like pieces oils. This is a room of bamboo walls in which there is a chest of drawers for privacy. If the soul is not visible, and this feeling of solitude makes you feel calm and free. Your independent inner voice rises in the same way as in childhood. You can do whatever your heart desires without condemning and not scolding others when you enjoyed the time unattended. You turn on the shower, taking off your clothes, and letting warm drops fall on your face and washing away dry salt from the ocean and afternoon sweat, as well as dust and dirt. When you explore the islet, air builds up, and waterfalls through cracks on the wooden floor. You take soap and shea butter and soak it in your face. Your body massages it when you cleanse yourself and inhale its sweet scent. The soap creates a feeling that is washed off. When you allow your face to feel a cascade of water on you when you stand outside in the rain. In the summer night, you turn and let the water massage your back when you look at the Indian Ocean. Now a vast black mass with strands of silver made of scallop waves under the starry night sky, which you perceive in this luxurious sensation, so simple and rustic. Even more fulfilling and memorizing than in the most luxurious hotels. You turn off the shower, feeling like a chilled night breeze. When you take a towel and hide your face in it before washing off the remains from the body, wrap it tightly around your head, take soft linen, put it on, and put it on a belt around your waist. The fabric floats on your delicate skin, dancing under the light breeze.

When you come to the second set spiral staircases, your hand feels the slippery curved snags of the railing supporting it as you rise higher and higher. Now seeing the floor on branches and green leaves rustling in the wind lace, like the silhouette of the leaves of the bay. Bob moves very little to show the stars above you. You find yourself on the third floor of a treehouse surrounded by a four-poster bed, which is also made of driftwood and is surrounded by a white mosquito net, some of which are facing the ocean. A deck that protrudes above the water below. When you stand at the railing of the bridge, you feel like you are in the ocean in the middle of the ocean. When you look down at the dark waves under the crescent moon, which has disappeared silver-white since the sky is now midnight black. The stars twinkle on you, for a moment, close your eyes and listen to the rustle of trees and the unbroken ocean. You feel respect for the timelessness of this moment for everything that attracts your attention that existed long before you and will exist long after you leave. You feel like a happy passenger on this journey in time and space, divorced from any problems and anxiety.

Because they all seem so small and temporary in the light of everything that lasts as long as the Bayeux Bob tree, the Indian Ocean, and the crescent moon above, you are just a witness to the grandeur standing on this balcony overlooking the vast landscape beneath you. You make a conscious choice to remember this feeling and come back to it whenever you feel depressed or stressed. When you are tempted to open a box of problems and worries and turn to them, you may find that they no longer serve you and our best left alone because it helps you the most. It is a feeling and trust that you will also endure the fact that you are healthy and hardy and, most importantly. You have the imagination and can rethink the beauty of the Indian Ocean. You are interacting with the lemur and her child, like the sound of leaves rustling above your head. The energy of an ancient tree that offers you shelter and respite tonight. In this great state, you feel the inner calm, sighing, and approaching the bed. Push back the mosquito net and climb onto the high bed, allowing yourself to go under the soft cotton sheets that smell fresh and clean. You adjust the leaves around you and scream the mosquito net that you are safe and enclosed in an ideal capsule to dream of feeling so close to the stars that you can see above and around you feel safe on the bed. You are grateful for safety and comfort, knowing how rare this has been for those who occupied Madagascar for centuries before you. You feel so happy to be alive in time and place in history. If you are given such luxury, it will not go unnoticed for you this morning. You can spend time remembering all the pleasures and privileges that the progress made by innovators over time. Even at the time when the present moments that have warmed your heart give you truly reconcile with everything that will disappear in this life.

You realize what else will remain your imagination. Your inner voice is the thread of you that existed in time from the earliest memories and experiences to the present moment until you realize that one day you will understand that the more you keep your imagination open. The more you can dream of a life that satisfies you. The more you can quickly solve problems on top of a tree, hiding in bed between the ocean and the sky. You can drift and let go of gently swimming over the bridge to your dreams soft as a breeze coming from the Indian Ocean. Soft as the fur on the lemurs of a child. As sweet as your skin is after a shower in the open, the air is made with luxurious soap from shea butter. It is soft like the whispering of Madagascar, urging you to let go at that moment to see what is around you. You feel the softness of the breeze. The softness of the night, the softness of the pillows of sleep and peace and dreams that await you. I'm going to count you to a therapeutic and beautiful vision, filled with the idea that rightfully belongs to you. Which you deserve ten nine eight seven six five four three two one find liberation find peace find a dream it's time to dream.

Coping with Crisis

Get rid of anxiety and relax with the help of sleep meditation, which is designed to help you deal with the situation during the crisis. We cannot change things beyond our control, but we can adapt and change the way we perceive them. We can focus on self-care and start from the very strongest. The healthiest and best versions of ourselves, so find a safe and comfortable place. You can let go of all your worries and fall into a dream where you can offer yourself a feeling of love, gaining stability and focusing on what you now know that this too will pass. I have the resources to find the most effective ways to cope and manage: every night and every time you want to return. Now, as during this meditation, you can see how this feeling disappears and is replaced by a sense of self-confidence. Since the beginning of time, there have been crises that have affected the life of humanity. It is not uncommon. This is to be expected, the longer we get to learn love and experience things on this planet. Humanity can prevail, and you can prevail, using this moment as a reminder of your limited time on this planet so that you can remember that every moment is so valuable that you can feel gratitude for the essential things that keep you alive. Because tomorrow the sun will rise again. Now you are the life that you breathe, think, expect, and feel. You are going to take control of what you think when I guide you towards times. When we must isolate where we must protect ourselves, it's perfect for leaving and being the one who decides which filters to use in your life, having access to endless information and with the advent of modern technologies. It's effortless to perceive too much.

You don't have to know everything because you can set yourself up and decide what you need to accept. Perhaps sometimes our ego tells us differently, and we resist the search for peace. We are addicted to chaos, but we know that since you made this choice to listen to a connection with your higher self. You can find peace. It would help if you took the time to congratulate you on making this decision and make a choice in favor of making you feel better. In times of crisis, you should not focus too much on fluctuations from one moment to another. At the same time, every day, think about the broader picture of the progress that will happen in months and years about the development that comes from a considerable period. Let go of any judgment or expectation, and when it should end, because it will end, like all things, and just like a photographic filter. You can change your perception and how things appear or feel based on what you, if necessary. You can always tune in to good in any situation. You can decide what information to accept and determine what is best for you today and tomorrow, starting right now. As if you had a remote control in your hand. Now I can give you a remote control that you can visualize in your hand, capable of changing your mind's programming. What beautiful images you would like to see if the remote control was used with care? Banaz, you go to this beautiful place. You can imagine that your room is a safe bubble that surrounds you and protects you before you go into a deep sleep at night. You can imagine that you are safe to go deeper and deeper.

You are free to be the most authentic version of yourself. If you need to cry, you need to take a deep breath. If you need to shake your body and the last impressions of a hard day, you can do it without shame or judgment is a zone free from experiences. You can freely express and feel how you feel. But these are not emotions, but reality. You can find the distance between your reaction to fear and the reality of what is happening at the moment. You can take these unforgettable impressions of the day and change the channel right now. When you take a deep breath, letting your whole body begin to expand. When you fill your lungs to the limit, like a balloon, you can feel lighter and be able to sail before exhaling and breathing in all this, angering you back to your bed, feeling the release breathe deeply again. Then exhale that you're beautiful, you're fine. The most important the tenant in all this movement feels the confidence and stability within himself. Feel that you have the inner armor that notices it right now, protecting your torso and giving you the inner strength, muscular and elastic, lively, and in the season. When all crises pass, and all trials can have an expiration date, nothing lasts forever. You know that this is true, and in this truth, you can find peace until life unfolds as you would like. It is better to take control of what you can. Indulge in something that goes beyond your control, like a sea turtle that glides along a wave floating with the stream. So you can feel this fluidity right now, imagine that it's sensible swimming on warm turquoise waves under the radiant heat of the midday sun smells of saltwater. The hat rolls over you like silk, supporting you.

At the same time, I was gently shaking you. While you are swimming, you control your breathing with deep breaths that exhale Bob's tide. The same is in your current situation if you fight the course or fight. You can create more danger and become more exhausted. But just letting out the floating without stress, you can survive. Because many strong swimmers could not escape the Riptide, fighting it. Therefore also surrender so that depending on your circumstances. You can only do what you can, and choosing to let will save you the strength to find the solutions you need when the time comes. The night of restorative sleep will help you. The battle for you is a warrior. Sometimes you may need a magic wand to take away all the pain, contention, and frightening thoughts about what might happen. Still, anxiety is just a projection; not your mind is trying to prepare you. When you prepare for sleep, you can make it clear to your brain that rest is the best solution; sleep will strengthen you, restore you, and allow you to accept all the challenges. This can happen because right now, it's just for sleeping. It's a beautiful, intoxicating feeling of liberation and relaxation.

You can rest tonight by focusing on what is right now. You are safe now. You are alive. Are you steady? Being with a verse that came to your body and your life without any expectations or worries, you were only you. You can return to it right now by visualizing a remote control in your hand that can control your mind's images. This remote control does not look like any other remote control that you saw before it glows as if it has its aura and your favorite color. With it, you can project onto the screens of your closed eyelids, and you are glad to see that in this life in this world. This is what makes you smile and feel gratitude? To focus alone on the image that you just clicked on to see how lively it is? How happy you feel? Instant, but transferring your sense of smell is activated by this beautiful moment. When you feel real as if instantly moving. Your imagination fills the entire sensory memory, noticing sounds that notice the physical sensation of contact with this magnificent image. You can even decorate your vision, which has no boundaries. You can do it even more special and fantastic visualization of what you like, holding on to this beauty. You can visualize that you melt it all in a golden elixir. This liquid can fill the bottle that you hold between your thumb and forefinger, watching it flow into this glass jar, encapsulating this enjoyable experience.

You were then placing this bottle on the necklace to hang it on the neck so that the bottle falls on your heart center. You feel the heat that penetrates your heart center, like molten candle wax. In your waking life, you can remember this necklace by focusing on it every time. When you need to remember the beauty that exists in the world and the fantastic things that you can connect with. Because even during a quarrel and also in the most challenging moments for you. Your loved ones and society as a whole. You can connect with this feeling that you can raise yourself so that you are better prepared to deal with everything that you deal with. You deal with it so well that your thoughts and fears can be like the sounds of bells. Their frantic energy can afflict you. You can visualize every call in yours. When you stand at the base of a quarry, noticing how it seems that they continue to ring without your control. The water is deep and shiny aquamarine. You take each bell and drop it into the water, and it would seem a bottomless puddle the water receives the signals as they sink more profound, deeper, and deeper. These worries become more and more muffled as they go more in-depth, as pure water absorbs all energy and sound until everything you hear e is a light ripple of water.

Then the stillness in your mind complements this experience. Because the challenge mind and the prepared mind that spent the night of deep sleep are more ready to react and thrive in any circumstances. When you are more capable of being yourself, you are more capable get rid of it and activate solutions. There is always a solution to any problem to make your life easier. You deserve to make decisions with ease. You deserve to feel better and have common sense and imagine that your bed, in which you are diving, is now a nest. You are deeply rooted, as if high on the trees that are under the summer sky. From this point of view, you can see a more comprehensive picture, which you can see in the distance. The ocean, sparkling like diamonds under a starry night sky and a piece of the moon that you feel so close to the air. But in a nest on a flexible and robust tree that flows in the night the breeze. The tree knows when to give and take, and therefore, understanding how the wisdom of knowing when to give and when to take will guide you to everything that you want right now—allowing your thoughts to return to a safe place in the room where you are now comfortable and relaxed.

You can go outside yourself and, as if observing from the side, looking at yourself in bed where you are satisfied. You notice how calm you look, watching how your body breathes easily, breathing in exhale when you find the inside peace inside. I'm going to count you down to the moment of healing that awaits you, where you can become intense. Where you can prepare for everything that can come, where you will find healing ten nine eight seven six five four three two one to find bliss to find salvation to find relief to find a dream, it's time to dream away.

Falling Asleep in A Rainy Forest

Your eyes are closed when you drift in comfortable sleep. You can feel that someone who walks in everyday life wakes up, goes to work. All his life is polite to others, goes home, watches TV, goes to bed, goes to work. They were respectful of others going back, watching TV, going to bed. Every day it was their usual thing, not waking up, going to work, going home, watching TV, going to bed. Then one day, they woke up and thought that they didn't want to continue doing this. They wanted something more exciting in life because when they remembered their path. Only a few memories stood out, most of the memories blurred into one that they could not distinguish once. Then get up, go to work, go home, watch TV, go to bed so one day when they were at home. They decided to surf the internet and accidentally book a vacation wherever they were. To know where they just wanted to book something, and they scheduled a vacation in an exotic place. Suddenly when they were going to work. They thought about the excitement of this trip that they expect in the future. While they work and smile politely in there, they think about what this exotic place on the way home will look like, thinking about the holiday that they plan to continue, and looking forward to it. Every day they cross out the date in the diary when they are getting closer and closer to their trip. Then the holiday came. They went on that exotic plane, landed. They went to a hotel. They left their things at the hotel. They decided to explore, and so they went out, exploring them wandering in beautiful the rainforest.

The sounds of birds, the rustling of leaves, the sounds of monkeys in the distance, and all the other sounds that they could feel, how warm it was in the rainforest, their attention was so focused on the excitement. The study did their water at a distance that they pushed through the rainforest. The sound of the sea grew louder and louder. They continued to push through the rainforest excited, surprised at what they would find. The sound of the water grew louder and louder until, in the end, they didn't see themselves suddenly clearing.

The light from the sun fell upon them, sparkling on the water of a giant lake surrounded by huge waterfalls. They could see these vast waterfalls, splashes, and fog rising at the bottom of the waterfalls, and rainbows dancing in the water as it was sprayed over the lake. They saw something like a small wooden boat descending onto a lake. They went down to the boat, climbed into the boat, picked up the ore thrown off the board, and carefully went out into the lake. They felt the strength of the water on the oars when they sailed. They went out to the center of the lake. The lake was calm, only with these waterfalls around. But the water seemed to calm down quickly if it moved away from the water, and the lake looks very deep.

The man just pulled the oars into the boat, then put this backpack on the pillow. They lay back in the ship, only closing their eyes and relaxing, listening through waterfalls and the background, sniffing the freshwater air, feeling the subtle rocking of a boat on the lake, and feeling the warmth of the sun falling on them. They just close your eyes, take a few deep breaths and relax, only allow yourself to plunge into the moment. If they relax, dive into the moment when the sun continued its journey through the sky, gradually falling in the air. The sounds in the forest began to change from daytime music to a nightly sound and like a sunset so that a person opens his eyes and looks into the sky.

When they look into the sky, they can see a blanket of stars sparkling in the air of different colors. They can see the Milky Way stretching across the sky. They are destroying one point of light in the atmosphere now. When they looked at this point of life when they looked and looked, their eyes started to close again. When their eyes began to close, they opened their eyes open on the Red Planet, and, oddly enough, they did not have space equipment. They could breathe correctly as if they were just on the earth. Still, they knew that they were on a red planet, and they found themselves at the foot of a mountain range on Mars.

I thought it would be uninteresting to climb the mountain range on Mars. So they climbed the mountain, tracked the hill, and, going to the top of the mountain, noticed how they vibrate. It was red; they started to get a new perspective in this world. They sat down. They rejoiced at the performance, knowing that they were the first person ever to set foot here and like a little sunset on Mars. So that they could see two small moons in the sky and all the stars in the air that they could see in the distance, it will be the blue gums that they knew was, and they enjoyed either the Miracle of the gaze. This pale blue dot saw that all life on earth all known life in the universe is on this pale moon god. Suddenly there is a suggestion that life seems so fragile when all this is contained in this one place. Such a small area at such a distance and they felt love and compassion for this whole life in the sense it is essential to follow this pale blue point.

When the sun rose on another Martian day, thanks to this new knowledge, they descend from the mountain and, reaching the base of the hill, discover that their eyes open in a floating boat on the lake, listening to this water, feeling the warmth of the morning sun, they got the oars. They drove back to the shore, and meanwhile, they continue to explore the rainforest. That evening, they decided to pick up a tent for the camera in the rainforest. It was the tent that you pitched between the trees, which would be tied to the trees and kept a few feet from the ground. They needed to climb into the tent. They needed to be a few feet from the ground, and you would feel as if you were swimming. When they rest in the shelter, feeling comfortable and calm, they will notice how the canopy gently sways between the trees, almost as if it sways gently. They generously rocked at ten, and after a week of enjoying an exotic holiday, see colorful birds, seeing different monkeys. Another animal was taking many pictures and recording thoughts that came to mind. They returned home, and they valued their bed more than they appreciated it for a long time. They knew they should have done it more often when they rested in their bed, drifted comfortably, and slept deeply.

Healing the Wizard

It's a sleepy meditation on finding yourself on vacation, in a lovely house on a desert island. You will arrive by seaplane and then come by plane and pick you up at the end of the vacation. Still, while you are here, you are here alone. You can enjoy your own company, enjoy this island. You have the most beautiful beaches, warm sunny palm trees. Some other trees scattered throughout the island. In all directions, you look, everything you see is the most beautiful ocean, you can see the color of the sky. The island is small enough. You can easily stroll on it in one day when you relax on this island. You read some excellent books that you laid out on the sun, enjoyed some of this solar heat on your skin. You swam in the sea, feeling the warmth of this seawater. A few days later, you find yourself falling into the routine of what you do at different times. Waking up in the morning, maybe drinking in the morning, perhaps tea or coffee, juice, perhaps something else. You spent some time when you get some fresh air, relax, swim, stroll around the island, stroll around the island—just lying on a bed reading a book with an open window, with a pleasant blow of wind in the window and just the perfect amount of light. Then one day, you relax on the beach, looking at the sea, listening to the splashing waves on the beach, watching them roll, and watching how the sunlight sparkles on these waves? When they roll, noticing seabirds in the sky, just soaring there, orbiting overhead, maybe a random cloud.

While you relax there, enjoying the moment. You think that you have been there alone for so long when you notice the sound of steps and wonder. Then you hear that these steps are getting closer and closer, you put the book down, you look around you and see what you can only describe as a wizard. A purplish-red long magenta cloak is coming towards you and at the foot of the wizard, confidently walking next to this wizard, a little kitten. They two are approaching you. The wizard stops next to you. You just watched them cross, and the kitten sits down to the earth. The wizard says that your help is needed.

You don't know why your help is needed, but they tell you that your help is needed. They came here to receive you when you decide that you will see, you can help, and you will do what you can. The wizard says that he takes off his pointed hat fresh, puts it on the sand, and then points at the cap, and you look at the wizard with curiosity. They look at you, and then gesturing again and looking down at the hat. Then you ask if you want me to step into the hat. They admit that this is what they want you to do, and you go into the cap and disappear. Then they come in behind you and disappear, and as soon as they dissolve the wizard's hand grabs, I'm in a hat and attracts it to extinction. You find yourself in a field next to a tree, and above this field, there is the most beautiful fog. When the sun rises, the wizard puts on his hat. You feel very naked because the wizard takes his cloak off his shoulders and puts it on his shoulders. You still feel a little bare. The wizard makes it clear that you can quickly find something that you can wear and begins to leave this field. The air is fresh and calm. The sky is relatively grey. It is only under the sun's rays, shining low in the sky, shining right under this grey cloud. The wizard leads you along a cobbled street where a horse and cart are waiting, does he open gestures for you to enter the horse's door and the wagon that door you enter the trolley sits on soft velvet seats, noticing small velvet curtains in the windows of the cart. The wizard leans in, the cat jumps on his hand, hangs himself on the side, the wizard raises his hand. The cat jumps into the front seat, and the wizard climbs up. Then he starts riding this horse and the car along this cobbled street down towards the neighboring city when you are sitting behind, bouncing in this cart, when it is climbing over the cobblestones, hearing the sound of the wheels.

The sound of the horses' still does not know what is happening but enjoys the experience with curiosity. After a while the cart stops, you hear the wizard jumping down. Then you open the door from which you leave this cart. You see somewhere that You buy clothes and the wizard explains that they will let you have everything you want to wear for free, they go to the store with you. When you enter the store, you notice that all the clothes. Where you saw the stars disappear. You continue to observe and watch, paying all your attention to this point in space, you find and keep, and then you notice that the star disappears. As soon as this star goes, you are repelled from the cottage and almost like in the flying pose of a superhero. You feel that you are flying as fast as possible to this point in space, not taking your eyes off where this star was. When you are very close to what was happening in front of the stars that you notice something like an asteroid. You adjust your course a little to go where the asteroid is now. When you get closer and closer, you see what looks a bit like a cave in this asteroid. You slow down at the entrance to this cave. Inside this cave, you understand that there is not enough gravity inside the cave to walk, so you think again that you have enough gravity to walk.

When you feel so, you find that the cape allows you to feel like a cape. When you enter this cave, it attracts gravity. After a while, the cave becomes too dark to see it and holding out your hand in front of you. You turn your palm up. You think you want light and shine. An electric blue ball of light appears above your palm. You notice the light dancing on the walls of the cave, your shadow dances on the floor on the walls. When you go deeper and deeper into the cave, and deep in this cave, you find the camera and it. In the camera, you have this feeling of movement on the back wall. You increase the illumination with this light, and when you do this. It illuminates the back wall, and you see the most beautiful moving patterns, symmetrical patterns dancing, rotating on this back wall, almost attracting you. You watch how these patterns move and change and again become one whole pattern. Then seem to take the form of several models when they move and change before becoming another entire pattern. The closer you get to it, the more You understand that this is more than just moving designs in which there are patterns inside patterns within patterns. The closer you get, the more repetitions you notice and the more. On the other hand, you find that what you look closely resembles the whole patterns that were even further, almost like a very similar model present at each level.

You come as close as possible, squint, and you try to look as close as possible. You notice that even squinting at the smallest scale. You can see the pattern that you are viewing inside the design, which was inside the models, looks incredibly similar to all other models. You feel that it is a little different, but if someone showed it to you. You would recognize it as the same pattern. With your other hand, you reached for the wall, put your hand on the wall, and noticed how your hand was getting closer and closer. Finally touched that wall, that, despite all this movement. It was not a physical movement, but you couldn't feel anything through your hand, fingertips, and palm. Yet, you could see that this is happening in front of your eyes. Then you noticed that something changed when your hand touched the wall. So the patterns began to change as if they came out of your hand, now copy your hand next to your hand, just slightly out of alignment with your hand, and then next to it.

Next to it, when your hands get out of your hands. These hands get out of your hands until the entire wall is full of replicated drawing that looks like your hand was repeated several times at different scales. Still, no matter how you enlarged it, it resembled your hand. You felt like you were standing between two mirrors and zooming in on the camera on the image of yourself in the mirror. You will see yourself behind you for an indefinite period, and, reducing the scale, you continue to see this wobble and movement of yours. You were behind you. You found it incredibly exciting since this wall seemed to turn things into patterns that you cannot explain. That the models seem to be moving, there seems to be some energy. Then you hear the bird tweet and hear something flutter. Then find a little yellow bird that lands on your shoulder and begins to tweet in your direction, almost tweeting in your ear. You get the feeling that he is trying to tell you something.

Then you understand that he is trying to communicate, what you need to go through it. You should solve this as soon as you focus on your hand and see how the drawing develops out of your hand, how it moves out of your hand. You begin to slowly and carefully move your hands, noticing how the entire wall of the picture changes and shifts. Then at some point, you get your grip so that the patterns across the wall suddenly synchronize. Suddenly look perfect and symmetrical. You hold. Your hand is in this particular place. The movement stops while it is in this specific place. Then the wall seems to disappear, opening into a dark area when you enter this dark space. In this mysterious space, you lighten this light in the other hand. You continue to lighten it and lighten it. In the end, it becomes bright enough to illuminate this area. You notice that this is a vast space. In the middle, it looks like an ancient well, and you go to this well. The closer you get, the more you hear a light dripping from this well. You lower the bucket into this well. You understand how it reaches the water, then lift this bucket, look into the bucket and see this glowing electric blue water. You touch the water with your hand and suddenly all this space, almost like someone else's picture in this space.

In some wavy film turns into a vast meadow, you quickly hear the sounds of birds appear. You feel the breeze on your face. You notice that the whole city is down there note that this is the meadow you are in when you first arrived in that city, that you are in the same field, only now the weather is better. The sun is bright. It's like the most beautiful summer day. You can see that someone was sitting down on the ground by the tree; you are heading towards this person by the tree. You can see that he looks a little lost in thought as soon as you sit next to them. At first, your nothing don't say, sit there. You will be present. Then, after a while, just present, you will see that they begin to come back here and now and see how they start to move slightly. Then open their eyes, and this goes to you. They are not amazed to see you there. They are you. We know that you were there. They did not pay attention to you. You are just something that was part of their environment around them, while they are in another place in their mind. You notice a certain sadness in their eyes. You ask them if there is anything you can do to help. They explain how they lost control of their forces. They had to isolate themselves here to try to protect everyone that people think of whether they start to do bad things with their troops. Still, they weren't for some reason. They lost control of their forces, and you understand that this is the person you should help. You thought that you should help them in the morning. They explained that it was morning, but now they are far away. You are sitting, talking to them and listening to them.

When they talk about how their thoughts are distracted, their ideas are so focused on other things that their body is almost ceases to cope and begins to make their own. Separately from what they wanted it to do with his mind. You know that one thing you got is the ability to focus the mind on comfort on the curiosity that can drive where you want to drift. Therefore you say that you will help them gain control of their mind and body. So ask them to close their eyes, take a few deep breaths and begin to relax. When they start to relax, you will count from ten to one on each. Consider that they can go one-tenth of the way more profound in a relaxed and focused state of mind that will help them begin to gain control of their mind and body. You can have this feeling almost like a tree with which you are next to open, and you discover the doorway and some steps. You follow these steps deeper under this tree when you follow the countdown deeper. All the more relaxed in your mind when you learn to focus on being here and now at the moment. You notice their hands begin to relax.

You see, yes, their breathing deepens and relaxes. You notice how their facial muscles smooth out, how their eyes open to dance slightly under the eyelids. The stillness in their body, feeling that their hands are getting heavier than six five four three two one, finding yourself at the bottom of those stairs, when you enter the room and see a chair. When you rest in this chair, you notice that you are starting those who go deeper and deeper. While you go deeper, it's a bit like getting into a virtual reality machine where your body here in this chair is still calmly relaxed. Your mind is focused on inner healing curiosity and works on the areas that you need to go through, directing them through the experience of internal work in healing. You can see how they are sitting in front of this tree. You can see the signs by which they follow, drifting deeper, healing themselves. They experience this experience of being in this chair. Their mind wanders through fantastic and sometimes unusual experiences which they take and follow with great curiosity. Each experience deepens and heals itself through its mind and body, making all the necessary changes. You know when the right time will come to tell them that they can begin to return to themselves under this tree because you notice a slight change in skin color. You see a small change in the way the eyes move under the eyelids.

You notice a slight change in tension in the hands. A small change in breathing, and then you let them know that they can take as much time as they want to come back here. Now under that tree for the next minute or so.

36

You will give them that minute of silence to take as long as they want to come back here. Not under that tree, and then when they are ready, they come back. You see their radiant smile when they open their eyes. They let you know that they feel the world, a sense of harmony through their mind and body. They again think about this connection between their thoughts and actions. They share with you the healing that they have experienced. They thank you for your kindness, your compassion, for the time you gave them, for your support, for your willingness to share your knowledge with others. They tell you that they will be fine now and that perhaps you should go and find yourself. You are wondering what they mean, and they say that maybe you should go and find yourself in this cottage. Therefore you are slowly walking through the meadow along which you walk along this cobbled street you see people running around the city. You walk past the shops, walk past the market. You see a curious person selling potatoes at the market. You walk along the side street. You find your way to the lane that you walk along this lane. You see different birds flying in the sky.

 You see what looks like deer in the fields. Then you realize that it seems that the front of them is people. They just gather and chat when you notice that the sparkling ones come from this direction. You think that you see other things there. Then you hear a pheasant and watch it take off into the sky, flapping its noisy wings. You arrive at the cottage, enter the cabin, go out into the bedroom and the bedroom that you are surprised at seeing yourself lying on this bed, looking so calm, so relaxed. You are curious because you feel that you are you. Yet you can see that you are there. You do not want to bother them. You feel almost like it would be harmful to fret that you sleep there, but you carefully touch your head to check. You notice that your hand passes through you. You understand that it's you. You are almost your projection, like an astral projection or a projection of your consciousness.

Therefore you rest on the bed, sit on the same line with where you are lying. You rest, lie down in yourself and feel light movements. When you settle in your body, and you feel so peaceful, calm, and relax. When you notice that you wake up and feel as if you are crying and feel the experiences that you experienced, going down. You do something to eat. You hunt in the cupboards finding in a cupboard under the kitchen sink looks like there is an almost secret world there. But you decide that you have enough mysterious worlds. But for now, there are only so many secret worlds that you can visit only so many different dimensions to visit for the day and as the day goes on. You hear a knock on the door. You open the door. The wizard stands there with a kitten standing on their shoulder. The wizard says it's time to go. You did what you came here, and the wizard happens on you go back to this horse and carts, you go through the door to the back of the wagon. When you go through this door, you find yourself on that beach and turn with curiosity because it happened so fast that it happened in an instant. The wizard and the cat stood here on the beach with you.

The magician takes his cloak, thanks to you for your help, and says that you do not have time to relax. You continue your vacation, enjoying swimming in the sea. You notice a giant the first ray of manti. You plunge and swim peacefully with this ray when it glides across the ocean, just like the sun glistens in the water. You continue this vacation until the seaplane arrives to take you home. You go home back to the mainland on a plane. You go home to the end. Still thinking about the experience that you had on vacation, and when you return home. Let yourself take a post, put it on the side, drink a drink, put your suitcase back in you the garden. You see a small yellow bird at a drinking fountain. You will recognize it as a yellow bird from your experience. You are curious that in the future it will become clear what kind of experience it is and what it means for the present and will you ever see.

Then this wizard and cat again that night you sit outside, looking at the stars, watching them twinkle in the sky, watching the random shooting star. Before you go to sleep, settling down and drifts and floats so peacefully, sleep so comfortably. Sleeps well and deeply cures the most beautiful dream at night.

Moon Dream

You cross the bridge between your waking and sleeping life. This meditation will remain active even if you fall asleep, helping to paint the canvas of your dream landscape. So find a safe place to feel comfortable and allow yourself to plunge into a comfortable and relaxed readiness to begin. In this, let's say space, your eyelids can become burdensome for your tired eyes. Like the dark shadows closing on the windows, your eyelids block the light. They indicate that it is time to settle for a night breath when your stomach rises gradually. Your chest lifts clean, clean air, oxygen that travels through your body and exhales the heaviness that you possibly hold in your body, when carbon dioxide is released from your lungs and breathes in again, feeling this lightness in your body. As if every breath of air could allow you to swim, preparing you for this sense of being freed from gravity in a space adventure.

This expiration again releases all the burden and thoughts racing that you are no longer attached to the image right there. How would you feel, just taking off and breathing in as deep as if the oxygen you are taking could easily make you swim to the night sky like a balloon with helium in a cool evening breeze? When you exhale, letting go of everything balanced. You feel that you can move farther and farther from your worries. Your bed to the expanse of the Milky Way stars twinkle across the velvety blue-black sky. The silvery moon is full and high. You go deeper and deeper in the same way inside you will soon travel deeper and deeper into space, finding the stillness that is within you. So lucky now that you are connected to all the symbolic forces of your mind. This expansion of thought, this openness to all magic in this world, makes petty worries. Which sometimes can be repeated, like spoiled notes, seem even odder necessary because this inner connection with you and everything that surrounds you in this vast boundless space expands the possibilities. Note that now, when you relax in the back centuries and act like movie screens. You see your legs landing and bouncing on the dusty silver-grey surface of the moon. Your body feels floating. The light is decorated with a metal suit that protects you from those elements that you lived on the moon intending to explore, study, and participating in a new initiative.

This initiative is exciting and significant, and you feel tingling under a protective suit, causing goosebumps and a warm stream in your heart center, there is energy like lava. This feeling makes you smile under your space helmet. The fact that you are alone now, delving into this majestic moon, smiles to yourself, even causing the slightest outburst of laughter that comes from your satisfaction, to shake your ribs. With each step you feel limitless and seem to bounce off the trampoline, each step is like an ocean wave. You take the time to explore how you feel in your life. Your suit offers this safety feature, your helmet, like a globe around you, which in addition to physical protection, gives you a starting point for imagining. It is like to have a layer of protection against negative energy, and outside influences resonate with your intuitive inner compass. Because in this solitude, there are little whispers and an understanding of what you like and what you might want to see, unfolding in this new and utterly foreign place, inhaling and exhaling the purest clean air from your tank. While you continue to see how you look at planet Earth? This planet you came from now is seen from a distance

Almost like a valuable sapphire blue marble egg. You do not have enough time to see how your dear the planet thinks about those times in your life. That you might have dreamed of a star or looked at a man on the moon whose face was formed by Mauria or the seas of the moon, arising as lava, cooled many years ago to fill the smooth surfaces of basalt rocks. That you can now explore without the lights of society. You swim through space in the rays of pure, luminous moonlight that reflects off the surface your suit and illuminates the particles of moon dust that fill the air, like the sparkle and confetti that you reach and raise the moon rock. Which seems to call you something that this rock invites and soothes, reminds you of the days spent collecting shells onshore on your home planet. You enjoy this exotic experience so far from the place where your life began.

This is the most remote place you have ever been from home. Even with such an extreme distance, you feel like talking and finding Acquaintance in an alien environment that surrounds you and thus awakens a reminder in you that you are wherever you go. But deep down - this is a feeling of inner confidence and everything that you have learned in this life. All that you have experienced and overcome all the tens of thousands of involuntary actions that your cells and body take to give you life. This has been happening all the time from the very beginning before the memories begin. You feel that you feel at home, because the house, ultimately, is inside you deep inside you. When you breathe in and out, remembering that you are a life that is aware that it is within your power and that you can give to return your attention to this magical moon rock. Which you know, crevices and craters this piece of the moon formed by lava. For some reason, these dark spots on the silver/grey rock begin to glow. Your tired eyes, looking at the helmet, that is around your head. They see that the words are still here, like a sparkling font, sparkling on your new one like flickering Christmas lights.

You will find a guide and mantra that will lead you through this otherworldly adventure, again staring at you and focusing on the words "To be motionless." In a state of deep silence, you will find that you are exhausted, despite the buoyancy that you experience with each step deep into the bones

42

and muscles. Due to your tiredness, a lingering heaviness arises. You feel that vines are sneaking up to your head, which also feels slightly heavy and tired. You look at the blue-green marble of the earth in the distance and send thoughts of peace and love to everyone else at home. You feel that waves of joy and hope that you submit will be received in the same way that the tides will receive guidance from the lunar phases—understanding how to deeply feel the connection and make it visible from the farthest distances fulfilled with your mission during the day. You continue to hold a particular moon rock drifts a little bit in his gloved hand until you find a hatch opening into your underground shelter. Hidden under the surface of the moon, the hatch opens automatically. When you find out that you are greeting it in your safety, like soft hugs. Again you feel this feeling that you feel at home and relax, going down the hatch in the elevator, which is very similar to the capsule that closes you, bringing you deeper and deeper, inhaling and exhaling. When you go downstairs and relax in a calm environment to protect the elevator, the doors open into a closed dwelling that has been fully decorated to suit your individual preferences. Say, take off your spacesuit and helmet, yelling the relief that comes with being unoccupied in this climate-controlled space. You can freely turn into your favorite pajamas that are clean, fresh, and neatly folded for you, just waiting, and across the room, your bed looks like on the capsule. It protects and covers everything like a pea pod, which is in your favorite color | your palette.

Inside this hotbed is a cloud that looks like a plush mattress and a blanket that is plump and attractive. So simple, welcoming, as if you can swim on it as if floating in the clouds. You feel tired and general heaviness. A sense of accomplishment that lasted for a long day and lived as much as possible every minute. How good it is when this sense of accomplishment becomes part of this extraordinary experience. So far from home to remind you of everything that you carry within yourself. You are your guide. Your beacon of light, your compass that focuses on your intuition. Your intuition can sometimes illuminate parts of your body, giving you the feeling of feeling good, and whatnot. The more you are in harmony with this energy, the easier your life becomes. Somehow in space, you will be easier to tune in to this guide even before you have all your life experiences and the knowledge that you possess now. You had this real roadmap to help. Maybe you forgot with time. But in the sanctuary of this underground solitude, you are entirely alive and remind how the moon directs the tides into the sea. So our intuition can guide your life by inhaling and exhaling. You will find the moonstone and take it with you, feeling how crooks and uneven appearance in your palm for a moment remind you of a coral reef. When you forget you go to bed, the lights of the room automatically begin to dim.

The stone becomes luminous. While you are saying the words "be calm." You put up with silence, screaming, so filling yourself with cold, clean air to fill your lungs with pure oxygen and filter it in this protective dwelling, like a drink from a tall glass of water cold spring water. When you lie down on the bed, you cuddle up to a plush blanket and pillow and allow your body to relax, feeling so comfortable and quiet. In this peace, you find peace. Reverential and serene coziness wrapped in a blanket that surrounds you, allowing your eyelids to fall on your tired eyes. Allowing your body to relieve any tension or hold a failed explosion for this magical. The otherworldly experience that made you feel even more connected with the world. You came from thinking about everything that you are now grateful for allowing thanks for this time allotted for rest, to bring you deeper and deeper into a state of satisfaction with his bliss. I'm going to count on you. You can even imagine that you smoothly travel along the silver bridge, which shines like the metal aura of the moon. The bridge is your path between awakening and sleep, stepping on this bridge, gliding forward, and bouncing freely one step by step to finding peace.

Night In Hoi An

Embark on a journey to Hoi An, a port city in Vietnam that has been greeted by a merchant and apprentice for centuries—now known as a romantic city where travelers come to do self-catering magical salvation. You can find yourself walking along with a kaleidoscope of silk lanterns strung along tiny chaotic streets, boarding a sampan boat, and riding along a romantic channel. The journey ends in the historic boutique hotel where you are before you escape to your luxurious suite for the night—living and staying in your body. You can feel yourself comfortably cuddle and indulge in this Mystical trip to Hoi Vietnam and any part of this vacation for the mind.

Everything in this experience should be adapted to your preferences and your needs as well as when you are sitting down in your bed. You feel softness and fluff on a baby, covered with branches with her brothers and sisters. The whirlwinds say to protect you, take the biggest breath that you can let your whole body expand like a balloon. Before you breathe out, breathe it in and breathe in like a newborn baby covered in a crib. Even heard if you want, and again take a deep breath, just stretching your body while it expands to the ceiling in your room. You can swim away and then breathe, doing as if you like. Since you feel good right now and for the last time, let your breath turn into a big yawn. You are now free to yawn whatever you want, without judgment from yourself or others. This is your happy zone, free from experience and back from your heavy, tired eyes. You can see how your feet are stepping onto a cobbled street in the old city, where Vietnam is decorated with sandals. Your fingers are free to enjoy the fresh air of the late afternoon. As the vibrant minerality of the river creates a wet fog of this river marries the sea. It is responsible for the prosperity of this particular trading port, a historic village, for centuries you have been walking along crowded streets past markets selling exotic spices, fish, seafood, and fruits and vegetables. Such exotic ones that seem almost imaginary sellers to you. Stands at the table with dragon fruit, so that Nate looks like exotic fuchsia.

He offers you a slice of his salad to try, which is crispy white speckled with black seeds and feels like water. You will feel the hydration on the lips with a more delicate aroma, and you feel relaxed. You feel the presence at this moment, even in the chaos of the market and on the streets that are crowded with other tourists and locals. As scooters weave into and out of the crowd, like a ribbon interwoven into a strand of hair, you feel alive. Your inner peace of mind activated in the sounds of people laughing at spinning engines and a stray dog barking. You feel at one with everything around you are in this distant country, so far from home. Yet you feel as though you are still with you because wherever you go there. The temperature begins to decline as the suns start to set on the opposite side of the river. You go down to the Riverwalk. Local Vietnamese men catch fish dangling over a ledge. Boats lowered to the shore, painted in bright shades of royal blue, orange, and dark orange, their colors fade on a dirty forehead. In a river rich in minerals, small Vietnamese children jump from one boat to another and then run along the path.

You giggle all the time. You recall this universal feeling that children played when the future was unknown ahead. You can be stupid for no other reason. It seemed natural, and it was good. So you continue on the path back to the heart of the historic old village. There are pedestrian bridges that connect both sides of the city, and the sky becomes lush purple. The river, teeming with whirlpools of thin white clouds and deeper shades of maroon, reminds you of a raspberry cone of soft ice cream, rushing endlessly past. Where eyes can see the end of the river before it joins Vietnam, seeing how you walk along more to the old Vietnamese, ladies with lines passing through their sun, whether they come across this as a road map from everything that they saw in this life, offer trips in their backpacks. Which these small wooden boats begin to fill the waterway with other travelers, as the day approaches towards the end of the woman. They turn to you. You decide to board her small boat to ride. Her eyes are so kind that they express a willingness to contact you, even if you do not speak the same language. There is still understanding and her steady hand ability that she begins to grow in the heart of the canal. She looks regal as her hat without a law in her traditional cone shape creates a startle linen silhouette against the background of bright colors of the fiery sky and brightness.

In the history of this beautiful country in which her fortitude lives. The story is told, and the spark of her persistent look forward, she guides you under one of the pedestrian bridges. It would help if you bent down so as not to plug your head. She laughs at you playfully, Vietnam. You need to pay attention and pay attention to what you are doing joyfully and full of life. You close your eyes for a moment, enjoying swaying back and forth in the gentle waters - the kind captain whispers to himself, from time to time, talking with his navigation friends in other Sam's pots ways. While she hugs you, Pat, making it clear that you can relax with his gentle motherly touch. Her strong hands are gracefully plunged into the water while you continue to ride your sleigh in a comfortable, relaxed, holding the city, as now the sun has disappeared.

You open your eyes and watch the silk lanterns begin to illuminate the old town. As if all the shades and the most varied boxes with pencils are captured. As the silk lanterns rainbow like an array against the early night of bright red and purplish red, tangerine yellow and sea blue fuchsia and bright green light flare up on the ground. Suddenly the candles lick and release into colorful paper floats. It looks Pooping like open Chinese food boxes bordered by lace edges. Our Guide offers to sell you a few pieces, and you smile and agree that you choose three of your favorite colors. She collects a paper float and lights candles to give you at least the first candle as a proposal. Since it is a tradition of ritual and with sincere gratitude for those who appeared before you along the line that brought you here, you take the second candle and release it into dark water when you make a wish for those you love most in this life. Sending them the kindest beings from this mystical place, knowing that everything you wish will be felt no matter how far you are from them. Perhaps he watches this candle floating away, dancing on the soft pulsations of the way gracefully, like a young ballerina. Then you take the third candle, hold it near your heart center, and take a deep breath when your chest expands. You lower it into the water when Yes, exhale and make a particular desire for yourself, perhaps this secret desire that you kept to yourself, maybe this is what you wanted for a very long time. Still, I was afraid to admit it to others or even myself, but what would it be whatever it is, it is your desire, and you deserve it. Right now, you deserve to send it to the vast universe, allowing it to swim away and reflect in the infinite space that goes beyond the deepest parts of you.

Where you held a particular dream and nurtured it, your gentle leader smiles and begins to row this door. A parking place, you enjoy the rest of the trip as the water now becomes more festive thanks to these colorful floating paper lanterns that illuminate the entire waterway. My Christmas lights are pulled over a tree, and it gently leads you to the dock. You can take a deep breath, exhaling before rising, she reaches out her wrinkled hand with a firm grip and helps you raise your eye neat for the last time. You smile generously by tilting it for this unforgettable experience, how blessed you feel that there is a calm feeling in your body. When your muscles become softer, like the warm wax of candles of floating candles. You feel relaxed as if your lungs are released from the weight of the day. The stress that you sometimes inadvertently take on, now everything has passed. It feels so lovely to be in your body. You are along the water under the colorful silk lanterns that are reflected on the river, like a kaleidoscope mirror it seems you're inside tiffany a stained glass lamp.

Since the center of the old city is completely warm and full of bright flowers. You will continue your journey through the historic buildings influenced by French colonial architecture. Balconies on the second floor of this brightly colored row of buildings are restaurant guests enjoying local dishes. In the kitchen, you decided to visit one of these places. A young housewife welcomes you and leads you to the balcony on the second floor, as soon as you sit down. You order a particular local house and watch the decorative lamps hanging down and vary in a round shape from full to miniature and compact. Your food becomes soaring and hot. The fragrant aroma hits your nose when you breathe in and relax in your chair. The beauty that opens under you at night is a lie with joy and brightness, and it looks like a special holiday.

Although for many locals, this is just another night in Hoi An. You finish the meal and rise, leaving payment at dawn, going down the narrow staircase of the building. You feel that you went back in the 19th century, the smell of a wooden staircase, the interior reminds you of a saloon. At this moment, such an exciting mixture of history unites different cultures, and you feel their wealth. Go outside and continue towards your boutique hotel on the outskirts of the old city. Which you leave among visitors and locals, feeling how much you are doing here, feeling the magic that comes with traveling and experiencing something new. Still, familiar exotic and, at the same time, able to navigate. If you last look at the beauty of the river, listening to the melody of flowing water and laughter in the conversations happening around you in different languages. You understand how energy is transmitted without an accent. So spend this night talking with people in deep and catchy ways. Without saying a word, and it feels special. It makes you take note of the energy that you emit, just like multi-colored lights. At the same time, patterns, sizes, and fabrics can change the light that shines from the inside - this is which illuminates the night. You can continue to light that around you. You will come across marble steps leading to your boutique hotel designed by our Nate Lee. Tall white columns and white grilles on the edge of a bright yellow building. The outer walls are quite brilliant and beautiful, and you go to the hallway and past the reception desk.

Which Jade welcomes, who looks after you throughout your stay. She reminds you that the massage planned in your room will begin soon, and hand you a cup of tea. You will take a jasmine-flavored drink and continue to your room. You will go through the courtyard and the deep sapphire blue pool, which reflects the stunning full moon in the sky above the soft fog rolls from the river. In the yard, the night air fragrant from the salty swamp. You see, as the fog enters, like a spider web above the stars. This curtain of fog is empty, and that muffles and softens the night when it is profoundly sleeping. You walked to your hotel room and opened the door to find the entrance, aligned with the rooms. Still, directing you to a huge bathroom, the design is modern and sophisticated. A rain shower is installed in the corner, and the water massage therapist will meet you in the closet. A massage table was set next to a large shiny white bathtub, which rests on a bed of stone. The tub is filled with a free channel in shades of burgundy, and yellow candles are lit around the room. The masseur suggests that you undress and get settled on the massage table. When she leaves the office, you take off your sandals and clothe. But carefully hang them on the rear door hook.

Then carefully slide under the soft cotton bedclothes on the therapist's table comes back. It opens the wooden doors above the bathroom that allow you to look at the luxurious king-size suite. The suite is decorated with Vietnamese works of art and paintings of the local river and rice fields. It's convenient to sing them here, as she holds a selection of oils in front of you. You choose exotic ones and remind you of ripe fruits and spices in local street markets. She puts oil on her back and neck and begins to massage the tension points that you hold deeply. Her hands are strong, intuitively feel the places that need the most relief, and you inhale, exhale and let go. She runs her fingers as if playing the drum up and down the spine. You feel goosebumps occur when your body melts in the table, feeling more and more relaxed and relaxed, it massages your scalp. It tingles and feels so good in her arms that drowsiness moves like the fog outside, turning you into a comfortable numbness. The massage ends, the faucet is turned on. Freshwater fills the bathtub, the massage therapist helps you to write, and thanks. She holds out her hand so that you know that the bath is ready, his smile when she comes out, glides through your body into the warm waters of the plumeria.

They swim like water lilies, go deep into the bathtub, smell like eucalyptus bath oil. When you take a plush rag for washing dishes, rinse Hydrated massage oil your body, like jelly, allowing you to find lightness. The day was smooth and full of new adventures and connections with other people with the beauty of this planet. The richness of the history of Hoi An and with yourself, as well as the beauty of travel, how fortunate you are for the blessings and memories that you have created that will be last a lifetime, like filling in how blessed it is. This wave of gratitude gives you the last piece of energy to rise to wipe yourself with a large towel before turning into silk pajamas.

Which is your favorite color you walk along the new floor to the large bed that awaits you? The ceiling fan whirls, creating a light breeze and an ideal temperature for sleeping. You say to yourself under the covers, allowing the crisp, fresh sheets, and bedspread under your chin to smell clean, washed, dried on the roof of the hotel, and the shiny sun. So simple but so comforting, breathing in and breathing out that you are ready to let go. You can continue to explore all the amazing experiences that your imagination can cause; there are no restrictions on which you can travel and delve into the most vivid and enjoyable images right now. At the same time, I will walk you across the bridge between your waking and sleeping life.

Secrete Under the Castle

Your mind begins to wander. When your account begins to walk, your eyes start to close. Your breath begins to relax. You begin to sink into your mind, falling into your mind into daydreaming, relaxing, dropping more profoundly, and deeper into your thoughts. As of how you relax and dive deeper into your account, you get the feeling that you almost hear cutlery. The sounds of a restaurant in which you find yourself sitting at a table opposite to the one you love to enjoy food together. A note about that is your favorite dish with a smell. Fear of eating this dish to cut food, weight when picking up any food item with a fork. The feeling that you put this food in your mouth chew this food, giving off saliva, looking at the person you like to participate in a conversation with them, sometimes just listening. Sometimes talking and eating some food and maybe drinking with this food and feeling the of this drink. It passes from your mouth through the throat to your stomach.

In this restaurant, a background sounds around you, mumbling people speaking at the sight of the movements in the corner of your gaze of the staff walking around and people moving around the smell of food that you eat. The menu of the one with whom you smell the food that you are not going to eat. The staff takes her past you on the most pleasant evening. After eating you and the person you leave the restaurant, you go on a trip to the promenade and go down to the sand one beautiful evening. You are noticing how the steps change when you walk along the sand. Your feet begin to sink into the sand with each step. Thus the closer you approach the sea, the sound becomes wetter so that under your feet, it feels different.

Stands on a moonlit night with a loved one who waves softly rolls along the shore, hearing its sound. These waves falling to the shore enter and reach the beach at various points and again recede to see. Perhaps, the stars in the sky, able to breathe fresh air and enjoy staying in the moment here. Possibly the moon coming out and you can notice how the moon illuminates the surface of the ocean and dances with the waves when you like being at the moment. Then you two go synchronously with each other along the promenade and down a bit, enjoying the secret tunnel opening in the evening.

You decide that you want to explore the secret tunnel. Therefore you two enter this secret tunnel, illuminating the tube with a torch, noticing how light reflects around the walls. Penetrating more profound and deeper into this tunnel, hearing the way your steps echo through the tunnel. After a while, the tube turns around the corner. You continue to follow this tunnel, curious where it leads you. Then you find the stairs along which you go along this road. Climb up and see the exit from the tube, exit the tunnel and understand that you are in the secret part of the nearby castle. You two are starting to explore this castle. You are wondering who knows about this tunnel. You know that you visited this castle before and never saw this room. You leave the room and explore along the corridor.

There is no lighting in this part of the castle, so you use the torch to examine and find the most beautiful beds. You find cabins with the most beautiful furniture and the most comfortable looking places, and so you study. Then you see the spiral staircase, and you climb this spiral staircase, and at the top of the spiral staircase is the door. But this door seems when you click on this button, you press almost the switch and not the lever. The door swings open, and the light enters. You understand that you are now in the central part of the lock. You two go through that door, the door is closed behind you. You know that the door looks like part of a bookcase. You are trying to figure out how to open the door from this side, and after a while, you understand this. You believe that you need to lift one of the shelves partially. The door opens.

You understand that what you found is the whole floor of this castle. It seems no one currently knows that there appeared to be an entire floor of the villa accessible only through this secret door. That it was probably untouched for centuries. The two of you walk around the castle for a while, and it caught fire. You assume that no one is in the area now, but you know that some of the castle lights often remain.

So when people look away from the castle, even at night. They may notice that there is a castle and that the window lights help determine that there is something. You two decide to go back down in this castle. You return through this secret door, close it behind you, go down the spiral staircase to the bottom, and begin to explore the secret rooms. The first thing you notice is that there are no windows here, as in the hidden parts of the castle do not seem to t of windows. Therefore no one ever found it because if you didn't find a secret tunnel on the beach or accidentally opened a secret door. If you didn't know that this level is under the castle, almost like a secret basement to the castle. You two go into the most comfortable room, sitting on the most comfortable chair. You are communicating, enjoy communicating with each other, and in this quiet room, feeling peaceful and calm.

Then without thinking, you both feel so comfortable that you start to fall asleep and fall asleep. You walk through a meadow with long grass that smells of beautiful flowers meadow trees scattered across a field. The most beautiful sky, a light breeze, is catching your faith. You notice that it looks like coolness with every breath. Then you go through this honey. We feel this grass at your feet. Then you see what looks like a rabbit hole in the meadow. You go to this rabbit hole. You go and sit next to this rabbit burden, wondering if any rabbits will appear or not.

I doubt that this happens when you sit there. When you sit next to this rabbit burden, you drag your fingers along the grass in the meadow, feeling the ticklish touch of the green and palms of your hands, and between your fingers, choose a dandelion and blow through the top of this dandelion. Then you think that you see something faint green glow inside the rabbit hole. You reach it, but when you arrive, you start to decrease. With the experience that you continued and so you reach further and continue to decline also. So the points where you are the size that fits perfectly into this rabbit hole find an exciting experience. You go into this rabbit hole, noticing where on this scale the dirt looks so that the roots of the grass penetrate through the walls of the row hole. Your eyes seem to adapt so that the light inside the rabbit hole and behind the rabbit hole is a very ordinary wooden door.

The unusual thing in a regular door is that it is inside and the rabbit hole. You open this door, then go to the bright marble room, noticing how your steps change when you go from walking through the mud in the rabbit hole to walking around the marble echo. Asks you to wipe your legs because otherwise, you will stain this marble. Then they will direct you to the mat. You will approach the mat. You will rub your paws. You will feel that this experience is becoming more and more curious, and then they say, come on, hurry. You have where that is, and they are in a hurry with you. Then someone else comes and says that their role is to make sure that you are dressed correctly. They measure you by measuring your legs, your waist, your shoulder measurement, you rise. Then Hinda is blind, and you go out with some clothes that they managed to create specifically for you. You dress in these clothes. Then you are asked to follow this first-person again after them along the corridor through a more complicated door to the ground. In which you feel like you are in the garden, a massive palace with spruce trees, shrubs of the most beautiful flowers, and flowers people dressed for the party. You go up the steps, following the person down these steps from the exit down to the central garden. You go down these steps. Then go out into the garden, and people greet you if they know you.

You greet them in a way and the garden. You have holes that you have to go to the great oak tree. So you go all the way through the garden to the very end in the garden, so the big oak tree that you see is on the back of this card. A person is walking with you to this magnificent oak tree. They ask the oak tree to move your fingers along the edge of the tree carefully, so gently slide your fingers along the side of the tree. The door opens, and you enter that door, go down into this tree deeper and deeper underground. You perfectly feel that your hand here seems to glow and illuminate the path. As if you were following yourself more in-depth into this tree, going down deeper and deeper underground. At the foot of the stairs under the tree, you find another door through which you pass. You enter the room. There is a chair in this room. You feel compelled to go and sit and relax in this chair so that you relax in this chair, put your hands on your side, and let the feeling of relaxation spread throughout your body. When you sit down and relax in this chair. You allow your eyes to close so that you begin to experience about feeling a comfortably warm ray of light coming down from the crown of the head down through the eyes, face, cheeks down your neck to soothe and relax you. When this light spreads down you, relaxing the muscles of the neck, shoulders, arms, hands, and back.

The chest relaxes to the abdomen, as breathing becomes more profound, more relaxed, relaxing down the legs down to the feet, and then feeling so deeply relaxed. In this relaxed state, you feel like you are at a different time and in another place. Your eyes and seeing that someone was sitting there and explaining that they are as a guide. Their task is to induce someone out of curiosity to find them here, where they can communicate. They know that they are in the right ways to help them understand what to focus on. Which way to choose to help them understand some of the more in-depth lessons in life about how to get the most out of life. They engage in conversation for some time through curiosity before they feel that they close their eyes again. The light disappears and then open their eyes. They leave this room, finding the way back to the tree, going the tree passing through the party, making their way through the palace through the rabbit hole. They gradually return to rest at this place in this castle. They leave the castle and return to the beach through a secret tunnel, and progressively the experience disappears. We go to bed and allow ourselves to drift and Sleep.

The Barrier Island

There is a barrier island waiting for you. This is the refuge that pulls you to your heart, like an anchor tied to a sailboat. With it, you feel a strong desire. It protects you from the winds of distraction and anxiety. So they can drive like you make a bet on the house and relax and relax in a safe environment. This barrier island activates the magical and healing components of your imagination. When we can quickly and gracefully fly to the highest heights on the wings of our creativity, this lets the creative spirit fill our hearts and minds with hope and fun. You could not do so in your waking life, but now you can piss off everything unique. You experience life in your body and in such a way that only you fully understand.

Because you understand that you can use everything that flourishes and smears on your mental canvas. The feeling is right and adapts to the experience and peace of mind that you can take before falling into a hoarse dream. Where you can fight Allie to dream, you feel that your body is becoming cumbersome, as heavy as wet sand, under the undulating wavy ivory waves of an approaching tide. You can close your eyes and breathe in, focusing on the words that I eat and exhaling, focusing on the terms, letting go of the inhale the words that I choose, and exhaling the phrase. Profound stillness, letting go and finding the stillness.

In contrast, you inhale the ale for the last time and exhale. You are even allowing this sigh to turn into an intense torment when you let your body understand that it's reasonable to perceive this feeling of such tiredness and relaxation. When you are ready to embark on this sea adventure. You start digging your fingers in the pale yellow sand of an isolated beach loved by vacationers who returned to the stream of their daily life. At that time, as your salvation has just begun. You have a salt respite here on the threshold of the new season when the slightest breath in the wind gives a warning that the end of summer is near. You feel the salt crystals that I formed on your bare feet from the sprayed dried on your skin. The sun is approaching its golden hour when amber reflection waves are reflected in our interval even with deep sapphire-blue hues of the ocean. When a few gulls fly for the last time before dark. When you watch them, dive, plunging their beaks into dark waters. The crab runs along the sparkling sand of at a fast pace contrasts.

The calm, gentle stream of waves that you decorated in a linen dress that combines soft, neutral tones of beige sand and hope to see the grass that borders the beach. You feel lined with it in a tone of neutrality and softness. You continue to go east, feeling the setting sun on your back. This orange, purple ball warms you and softens the tints of the tidal pools. So that they look like reflecting molten metal, the solitude that you feel in connection with you in an inner voice offers unfiltered understanding and fulfill the purest of your desires—providing guidance. If you close your eyes right now and breathe in the salty, moist air, you can feel the salt on your lips, feel the hardness in your nose. Clear your throat and heal you when you exhale while listening softly to the flowing ocean waves crashing to the shore, yelling a light breeze. When your soft linen clothes are torn on your skin. Tiny granules of loose sand raise your legs with a light peeling. You think that this calming mantra is here. You are so present, so associated with every sound, smell, and sensation. You are so connected with yourself, profoundly feeling how your body vibrates at a frequency of a calming tide and how you open your eyes? Do you notice how the sun has gone beyond the horizon? Small droplets of sea fog accumulate on your eyelashes, creating prisms through which you see the world around you profoundly inhales.

You exhale and find that you freely rotate your hands, enjoying pure bliss it comes with this feeling when your hands float like wings on a sea breeze. You continue to go down the beach to your house with an impulse of soft winds. When the sky turns dark, turning into amethyst, ruby , and earthen orange. You can feel the energy of the island that protected the mainland and was a refuge for a century of sailors who came to its shores. You look at the sea and observe how white ridges form further, where a sandbank was formed.

The waves gently flow in the shallow water, and the summer becomes soft, and all the sunlight falls. The hot temperatures also disappear and happen when in cicadas twilight begins to come, come to life with their little ones. You make your way past several empty snow-white beach houses. I am cleaned for a week. You seem to be the only inhabitant on the barrier island or a quiet evening. You notice how peacefully, and miraculously it seems that death - time only if you found this refuge for yourself.

You went to the faded wooden staircase leading to your glory. Who proudly stands on stilts protected from before rising, rinse your feet and hands with an external hose. Before washing off your face and tasting cold freshwater that cleanses you of salt and sand. After you carefully walk along each staircase. You feel soft, weathered wood under with your feet until you reach the main deck of this three-story house, go to the outdoor bar overlooking the beach. You prepare your favorite relaxing drink, have a snack before heading to the turquoise tree.

A rocking chair on which you can sit and swing back and forth. Continue to flow, take a bath, and back and forth, the chair moves like a path with its rhythmic flow, which causes comfortable relaxation in your body and when you are listening to the waves rolling on the sand in front of your beloved home. You can hear the whisper of leadership that is cherished and eternal. This barrier island has survived so many storms and remained intact as centuries passed. This stamina brought wisdom as if the sea were whispering to you that you are eager to hear eternal things and still within you. No matter how much time passes or roads, even if the shores of sand on this barrier island have blurred everywhere the time, when the energy of security and peace has always been restored and remained untouched by that side of the storm, like an island. On which you two have experienced so many storms that it seems too big to measure. You respect these shores that I met on swarms and swarms.

I traveled from far away, deeply understanding the relief that these fellow travelers experience. When they find land and take refuge on this barrier island. You feel protected by the misty brackish air that envelops you like a gentle hug. When you continue to sway in a chair back and forth, inhale and exhale the sea's whispers. I call you. You hear the words that you are healthy. You feel Wellness, which does not fill you to the brim. The center of the heart from your beating heart and lungs. Which are now filled with a cleansing breath, expanding to their maximum capacity, you do everything you need to do. Therefore you will learn from this whisper everything you need to do right now, everything you need to do it. It's a concern for yourself to focus on this inner peace, as the gentle rhythm of the incident waves leads you. The stars begin to lighten the velvety dark blue skies above the golden moon. Almost full and reflected on the dark silver crusty waters below.

You feel so pleased and so tired, so ready to find a place to lie down and sleep, or at night, and so you get up. You enter the sliding doors of your house. When your feet land on the cold ceramic tiles that we hand-painted and marine drawings in your favorite colors, these colors and images heal.

Your blurry tired eyes look like they turn into animations. These are watercolors when you watch bare feet walking on each tile, directing you to spite. Staircase leading to the second floor and continuing to count every step go one, two, three. You will take the high ceilings that open in the skylights and see the stars from above the comforts of your home. While she listens further, making her way through the wooden floors of the hallway to the master bedroom. In this room, you will find a bed with a canopy surrounded by transparent ivory curtains that dance under the soft ocean breeze that enters the room through open French doors. You go to the doors that open onto Juliet's balcony to enjoy the greatness of the sea. The last time you felt as if you were at the helm of the ship. You can drink every breath of salty night air and encapsulate this peaceful moment so that you can easily access any point you desire in your waking life. At any time when you need to connect again to suppress any anxiety about daily stress. We enter the room, feeling heavy and tired.

As the ceiling fan rotates overhead and makes the room relaxed and comfortable. You want to bury yourself under the crispy white cotton sheets and fall asleep. Although you take off your clothes and change clothes into soft bedding folded on the bed, smelling of fresh, clean linen, leaving the doors open for the night. You bend the sheets back and stand under them, talking. You allow your head to fall slowly. When it sinks into fluffy pillows that wrap around the curve of your neck and skull encapsulated like peas in a pod. You are very relaxed, feeling dense and dreamy. When the haircut curtains hang around hypnotic and making you feel sleepy as if their flying wings are about to fly away and allow you to immerse it in a healing dream. Where dreams can color your world with unlimited potential, still, now you look at the French doors and watch the sea continue to shine with a sparkling sea. You feel grateful, and you are striving for the natural rhythm of night and day, as from your internal compass. There is no time to direct you to sleep, inhaling, and exhaling.

When your heavy eyelids fall on your tired eyes, you feel so relaxed, feeling like a centering sensation arises. When you are at home, like an old copper skeleton key, when he starts laughing, creating the perfect pair, so what are you now? Say in your refuge when you find your perfect match, and by closing your eyes. You will feel the gentle rainy wind piercing your face, and listen to the ocean waves continue to fall. They come in and go out softly and soothingly, dictated by a full glowing the moon above you. You cross the silver bridge between your wakefulness and sleep. Where you can even lighten a dream, in this particular place, you can turn off my voice at any time. When you want to imagine that you can enter the inner curve of the incoming wave and safely find comfort in the seawater tunnel that is forming around you, imagining what it feels like to stay in the Center of this Path. When the deep sapphire blue color of its interior becomes about the moonlight's flickering, it causes the water droplets to form this path to be refracted and form a bright rainbow. That envelops you, and vibrant colors constantly swirl. When you dive deep into the sweet spot of this powerful path. You find balance. When you open the portal, it moves you to the other side. This other side offers you inner peace and tranquillity. It gives you a break where you can start dreaming. Where you can let go, let it all go right now, you are three more. Three lights and light-heartedness you are in the Purest celebration that you are allowed to be all that you are when you swim and gently drift to sleep. I am going to consider you when you will move deeper and deeper with each coat load and float to the best nap and most profound sleep. You may have experienced overtime to find the relaxation that ties immobility, find protection that binds you, find a dream world, and dream.

The Futuristic Home

Relax in this calmed time story and sleep meditation her stress relief and help with insomnia. A story will take you to a customized home far into the future. Where your home is an extension of you, it protects. You and gives you a sensation of serenity and deep ease. Before you drift to sleep, it's time to dream away as you get cozy and white down before sleep. Like that of your dear friend, help you visualize experiences that make you feel safe and content. Before bed, you cross over into the therapeutic world of sleep that awaits. You are free to connect with your imagination and set the tone for the dreams that await you. You may take in the deepest breath of the day, slipping in so much air that you could float away and sigh it all out. As you relax, make a sound and feel free in your body before you inhale again, taking in a deep breath and letting that breath fade into a tired yawn stretching your arms overhead. If that feels nice before you settle. Before you sigh it all out again, just letting go, and as you do, I want you to visualize that you are seated in a zero-gravity lounger in the back yard of your futuristic home. As you travel to this place, you can feel all the cells in your body radiating at a different speed transporting.

You to this perfect futuristic landscape, it is a time where the balance has been restored. At once, humans are at one with nature and technology in a way that every person on the planet is comfortable. As the world thrives, the change in humanity and on the earth is felt as you lounge in this chair that hovers above the vibrant green grass. Everything just feels lighter and more spacious. In this world, you can navigate the power of thought as it sends

---

66

navigational signals telepathically to your lounger. This future holds a world that is like a dreamscape where you just think and believe for something to come into being adorned and a soft cotton robe it cinches around your waist. The fabric feels buttery upon your skin; it is lightweight and breathes very symbolic of how you are now the crickets. Sing out on this balmy night as you float and relax your backyard is enclosed by a fence upon which vines of grapes and berries and tomatoes grow, in abundance, colorful glass mosaic orbs of solar-powered lanterns. Circle the yard in jewel tones of sapphire ruby and emerald green and create a warm and festive environment for relaxing beneath.

The Stars a fire pit is set a glow crackling within the confines of a sophisticated glass enclosure able to ignite. When you need it to your home is but a reflection of all the homes of the time. Where everyone can comfortably exist for the abundance that comes from a nurtured planet. You feel the delight of nature coming together with human comforts. As you look up to the sky, your home is built upon a rolling Hill among mountains and lavender fields that hint the night's air with a gentle fragrance. That lowers your heart rate and calm your disposition fireflies like delicate yellow dancing flames are cast against the plum. The black sky is a seemingly endless silver star. It's a knight of silver and gold when you most need to feel like opulence and luxury that has very little to do with material things on the deepest level. It has to do with the inner sensation that you think and the elevated mood that comes with self-care. The ability to feel soothed and tonight you feel soothed by the sounds of crickets and song by the balmy soft summer winds that blew through the valley. And create a subtle shuffle sound the comforts of the home are about an extension of yourself, and quite often, how we keep our homes is a reflection of how.

We are feeling inside inhaling the night's air; you feel a tightness in your chest. As you realize that you are free to think and contact whatever you want in a safe place. All for you, we're even self-judgment non-existent, and as you hover and float above the night's air, you go towards. A swimming pool that glows aquamarine from its inner light. You direct your chair to hover above the pool and then immerse itself. So you may lounge now floating upon the crystal waters. You notice the difference between floating on the water and the air; the sensation is more gentle. As the waves lap around like soft and races, you dip your fingers and toes around the loungers' edges. Enjoying the tepid silky water on this perfect night, realizing you have manifested and created the experience. All that is around, you must dream it for it to be looking to the Stars. You allow your eyes to become leery as you envision the galaxies far away. You feel small all your problems just as little as your butt one tiny piece of this majestic and infinite space it eases. You do know that you are supported and part of this vastness. Trust is instilled deep within that all will be okay and that all has always been okay. You go with a flow allowing the lounger to drift wherever the soft summer winds.

Take it before you bump against the edge of the pool and are redirected back to the center because life may always try to Center you and balanced you. If you do not resist, you may find yourself in this perfect harmony looking again to the silver stars. The golden glow of the fireflies, an outdoor fire, is a night full of twinkle feeling quite tired. You direct the lounger to the grassy area before the patio of your home. You disembark and walk towards tall glass sliding doors that open automatically. As you approach as you enter, you are met with a smell of home the scent that you most enjoy that elevates your mood and makes you feel relaxed. Perhaps the clean fragrance of lemongrass our eucalyptus or freshly baked goods or of flowers or other fragrance that conjures a deep sense memory. The home welcomes you in a voice that you have chosen, perhaps that of a loved one or of someone you admire. It's a voice that calms. You deeply as you are updated on the current time and temperature as the home wishes.

You enjoy the evening and relax because you have earned this experience. The walls showcase your favorite hues at any given moment with artwork that suits you. That is customizable based on your mood. So when you need serenity, the walls become marine colors of teal and sapphire blue and seafoam green. Just the same as when you need energy, the colors become bold and uplifting based on your thoughts and biometrics. You come into the main living area where there is a glass enclosure. That may transform into an indoor waterfall or erupt into contained flames based on what will make you feel best you choose what you need, and it becomes whatever that may be the ceilings are as high. Three times your height with glass skylights allow you to see the bright stars above in a design that makes you feel close to the night sky. The windows change their shade based on the amount of light you desire. So even in the morning, you may still sleep in as they are blacked out upon waking your biometrics. Allow the light to slowly pour in and awaken you at just the right time in your sleep cycle to feel wholly restored and refreshed.

In the main room, the furniture represents all that appeals to you. There is a massaging chair that you go to each night to relieve tension before it is time to sleep. You walk to this chair, taking a seat as you feel it hug around her body. As soft music begins to play sinking deep within the chair. You feel as knots of tension in your lower back and shoulders are massaged away with deep kneading and patting your body becomes soft melting like candle wax. As you go deeper into this moment of total bliss, a helmet comes down from the chair and surrounds. The crown of your head as thin strands of beaded metal weave through your hair and massage your scalp. It causes your entire head to tingle with a sensation traveling down your spine and through your arms. The backs of your legs, your body is covered in goosebumps. You feel they release you feel good and upon the most massive wall in the room images and videos play of your favorite memories. In this life with loved ones, your triumphs, and achievements pictures of things that you enjoy tampering your brain for happy thoughts. Before bedtime, the room smells now of summer with lavender reaching your nose as you inhale and relish. These memories, whatever memory you wish to recall, is projected. Before you, like a movie and connected with this home that is but an extension of you, it conjures other memories.

You may have forgotten the highlights of a life well-lived even when things. May feel hard. There are these moments to which you may always return whenever you feel stressed or whenever you feel down. They are the ribbons of joy that are interwoven within the fabric of all that you are, and you may visualize these illuminated strands flowing through your muscles, in warm sensations, and of hearing in lustrous hues of silver and gold. Because your body becomes more and more relaxed as these memories appear, as her body surrenders to the massage chair, you feel a tightness in your chest; your breaths are deep and comfortable. This thought comes to mind while I breathe. I hope each inhalation is another chance to dream and hope the massage begins to slow. As you feel a pat on the back and the helmet Rises, you stretch your arms overhead and walk upon the soft white floor of the room that feels. As if your feet are stepping upon a foam mattress massages the balls of your feet. As you walk and become a canvas for images, it also reveals the forest floor's calming imagery. Just like that, you're on nature's walk through your own home with all the sensations of being in a forest without the inconveniences. You feel safe in this moment of Solitude. You come upon a hallway.

It is another place that conjures sensations that you experienced at a point in your life when you think of a bedroom that was your most comfortable place to sleep. In this life, this experience or passes even that as this home is the one that makes. You feel the best that you have ever thought it is here to serve. You come upon the master suite as a door automatically opens. Then closes behind you, and it makes the room like a safe heart where you may find refuge and silence. The skylights take over the ceiling as well, so you may see the sliver of a crescent moon above the room urges—the beauty of nature with simple designs. A king-sized floating bed and clean white bedding the floor is made of bamboo. There is a bamboo wall on which orchids and exotic flowers grow in hanging glass pots. The room is sophisticated yet simple. You head to the ensuite and prepare yourself for a night of sleep. You step before a concave mirror that wraps around the bathroom sink illuminated with a soft golden light. The home assistant speaks to you once again in a familiar voice asking if you need anything farther. You then lift a mouth device that fits perfectly over your teeth and begins to brush and polish them for you with a minty paste.

You open a blue glass drawer beneath the sink that contains. A hot towel damp and French smell, so you take it and clean your face and hands as the automatic tooth brushing system continues to massage your gums and polish your teeth. You remove the tooth polisher as a water glass is automatically filled with fresh water. So you may rinse you catch your reflection in the mirror, noticing how relaxed and healthy. You appear your skin is vibrant, your eyes have a spark, you feel alive, and realize that even with all the conveniences of the future. You still feel like you, and you still have these human moments. You return to the bedroom and find soft, lightweight pajamas that you change into the room is dimly lit with soft purple lighting that makes you feel both sleepy. As if you're a part of outer space, you walk to the king-sized bed and pull back the sheets. As soon as you get in, the sheets tuck you in, and they are the fabric that adjusts to your temperature. So you are always most comfortable, and the air around you circulates naturally smelling of fresh pine. As if carried on a gentle breeze in a forest because, in the future, there is a constant marriage of nature and technology. As you get comfortable in the bed, all the pressure points of your body are adequately supported.

You look to the ceiling, and as the stars are visible through the glass skylights that occupy most of the space. The remaining parts of the roof become stars. As well, and the stars are connected to form words that have been proven scientifically to improve your mood. Boost your spirits, creating the proper framework for healing sleep. The first word to appear is believed scrawled in cursive above the fresh, comfortable bed. You think of all that you believe in feeling warmth in your heart and steadiness in your mind. Then the word dream appears, and you settle into a knowing that you will allow your dreamscape to give you guidance that may carry over. In all the days to come and may heal all the days gone by, and the next word that appears is love. You feel the sensation of love self-love and respect for all that is around you gratitude is abundant. The nurturing source enriched earth upon which a garden of prosperity. May grow, and the stars on the ceiling fade to black as the windows above begin to darken. You are in the safe pod of your bedroom. The circulation of the air of the master suite continues to emulate a summers breeze. As you inhale and exhale, feeling tended to and say as the nurturing voice of your home wishes. You a good night acting as a concierge available for you whenever a need arises. Just as there may have been a night as a child when you realized you're being nurtured and cared for perhaps even time.

As an adult and you rest knowing that the world of the future has restored serenity and peace in the homes. All there is a balance between mother earth and the advances of humanity. There are a balance and shift within humanity where everyone has a purpose and knows it and can pursue their best life and happiness in the Odyssey Homer expressed. There is a time for different words, and there is also a time for sleep, and whatever terms remain sounding off. In your mind may now come to silence as it is time for rest you have earned it. It is yours and comes the morning, and the Sun may break through the skylights above, gently easing you in a new day. No matter how much sleep may happen, you will feel refreshed. You will feel well I am going to count you down to the restorative and beautiful dream-filled sleep. That is rightfully yours and that you deserve ten nine eight seven six five four three two one finding release. He's finding asleep it's time to dream away the excellent night.

The Costume

Fall into a magical sleep tonight in this festive sleep story that will allow you to explore different empowering parts of your personality and spirit. You are listening to the costume, a mystical experience that will enable you to try three different costumes. As you are transported to various locations throughout the evening, that will provide you with healing strength relaxation, and joy. So take this time that is just for you to explore all the secret parts of your cell without judgment or interruption. Every day of our lives, we dress for different situations and use our attire to reflect different parts of our personalities. We play so many roles in this life that even the simplest of the dress is still like a costume. We use to empower us through another day and layout another role tonight. In this guidance sleep meditation, you are free of limitations on what you may wear and adorn yourself. So take this time now to settle into your bed, get cozy and deeply inhale and exhale, letting yourself go deeper and deeper down and within loading into a relaxed state. Your mind is a blank canvas upon which you may visualize all that makes you feel most content. At ease, I am here as your guide and Ally to soften your transition between your waking and sleeping life.

You may use the sacred time to dream and to recover from yet another day in this body another day into your journey. As you and you may let go of any thoughts of the day as we go through a brief breathing exercise, I invite you to visualize words that appear in the sand designed. In your unique handwriting and as you inhale, you see the word release appear within the reflective white sand. As the crest of a tide comes in towards you and as the white crest of the wave pulls you out, exhale. The newly washed Shore reads the word me and again inhaling you take your finger and drawback in the sand. The word release and then the warm healing tide comes and goes as you exhale and reveals—the word me just one more time drawing the word release. As you inhale watching the wave come in as you exhale, it goes out to reveal—the word me and whenever you feel stressed whenever your thoughts feel beyond your control. You may remember this. You are in control of your breath. You are in control of your dreams, and you may just utter the words release me that you may find yourself published failing heavy. As you sink into your bed, you may find yourself traveling to a different sea in your mind.

In the sea, it is a crisp cold night where the velvety sky Appa is bedazzled with silver stars that glitter around the moon's smiling sliver. A soft refreshing breeze hits your face as you find yourself walking on the pavement of a familiar Street where the street feels like home. It always has perhaps this was or is your address, or maybe this is just a street that you associate with feeling like you are home. Maybe the road is one to symbolically up here in your dreams. There you are walking down this welcoming street as an occasional car drives by; otherwise, the street is quiet. You welcome the solitude, and as you walk, your feet almost feel like they are gliding along. As if gracefully ice-skating upon the pavement, you look down and realize you are adorned in a costume that you associate with being safe. It may be ornate you may be dressed as a character from a favorite show or book, or you may even be just adorned and clothing that, like a cloak, feels warm. Protective against the cold night air allowing your imagination to take full rein. You let yourself go thinking to yourself, release me. So you may be released from any inhibitions our logical thought because just like in a dreamscape.

You now abandon all critical thinking and allow the emotional tide and sense memories to bring you this beautiful moment of exploration. You are taking this time in the center of the street that feels like home. You close your eyes and gently sway back and forth, feeling the glory of being in a body. In a motion that is entirely a lie and fully invested. In experiencing the present moment inhaling and exhaling. You explore the sensation this costume of safety for as long as you desire. You are taking note of every thread every color every stitch and every feeling that comes with the freedom of being on this street. That feels like home because when you feel at home, it is like a key put into the proper ignition enabling you just to turn on to connect with your intuition. The inherent powers you were born with the intuition that is there to guide you and coax. You through this life towards all that you so desire and with that as if an observer of your cell. You take a mental image of yourself feeling comfortable. In this costume of safety on the street that rings, you warp beneath the limitless stars. Above and you close your eyes and hailing release and exhaling me.

As you are transported now to your favorite room. This room may be anywhere. It may be a room. You are so familiar with what is perhaps a room that is entirely designed by your imagination to suit what you need at this moment. This room inspires bravery. You take in the decor the silence of the room. The sanctuary that exists here for you to dream and inhale the fragrant air the carries and aroma that you instantly associate with this setting even with your eyes closed in the deepest of silence. This familiar scent is like instant teleportation to a particular time and place in your life. Where this room has served you well even if the time and place are only right now and on the wall. There is a full-length mirror that you approach and take in the second costume of this transformative night. You are currently in a tire that inspires the feeling of bravery, whatever you are wearing this wardrobe makes. You feel empowered to overcome anything that comes your way. You are strong; you are resilient; you are aware that there are fears that will always come up to be afraid is to be alive.

But you are also given the tools to be brave in the face of all that scares you because you know that everything is temporary. This, too, shall pass no moment shall last forever. Your lips form a relaxed and tender smile as you look to the mirror again, lifting your arms, letting your body move in any way. That makes you feel free because when you are brave and free, you are unencumbered by the fears that hold you back from what you most desire. Often the concern we have come because we care so much because what we want is the right insight. We may be afraid to claim it but in the safety of this room finally. In the reflection in this mirror, as you find your body swaying and flexing muscles. Failing your own internal and external strength, you see a glimpse of your future where you are brave and seize and take what you desire to know. You may think of this room where your bravery was more and embraced in a tire that allows you to explore that side of yourself, whenever you feel timid whenever you are afraid of holding back. You may imagine being brave pretending for a bit even if you must because eventually, your mind and body will accept it. You will prevail you will succeed you are brave again you inhale and exhale feeling the clothing as it touches your skin. This costume empowers you one last time and leaves a lasting impression of how strong and how lucky you are for this time to pretend just like when you were a child.

Before society or adults affected your imagination and caused constraints right now. All those constraints are gone. They no longer serve you. In the privacy and sanctuary of your mind and in the dreamscape to come, you may Behe and dress in any way that suits you in any way that feels right catching. The reflection of yourself one last time in this costume of bravery, you think the fluidity of your body and motion. As you inhale and exhale on the words, release me and find yourself transitioning telepathically to a new setting. You are now in your favorite location, and you may find yourself longing to be all the time. This is the place that makes you the happiest, a thoughtless bliss that radiates. Through your body and allows you to be so content to be alive. This is a place where you would be all the time, but for the fact that the rest of your waking life experiences make this place all the more special reflecting on memories. That you had in this location, you are tingling with a warm sensation from head to toe as if goosebumps are covering your skin with the exhilaration. This place conjures wherever this place is. You may have a lifetime of memories that come to life like a film. In the early days of Technicolor, highly saturated and vibrant and whimsical and happy.

You inhale and exhale feeling the aliveness in your fingers, and in your toes, you feel timeless. As if time is not linear at all as if all these moments exist all. At once, this location is for joy, and so you find your cell adorned in a costume that makes you feel joy. You are dressed in a wardrobe that makes you feel a sense of fun and playfulness. The kind of outfit you would have chosen first if given a chance to dress up and play pretend from head to toe. You are the embodiment of bliss and profound happiness. Each breath is a tender sigh with the same contentment that comes after having a big, fulfilling meal or energy exertion. When dancing until you can dance, no more just sighing, letting it all go, you feel free you feel you can do anything laughter comes to you as quickly as it did. When you were a child free to giggle and relish at this moment, your laugh is like a sonic wave rippling. Through your cherished place that exists eternally, whether you are here or not, it is always within you this respite for the joy you deserve to feel happiness. The pleasure you deserve to relish in the Bliss that has been awarded to you like a blissful meditation where you feel liberated by our beautiful attire that makes you feel so special. So cute and the embodiment of a cherished life, you are welcome to invite in friends or loved ones who have experienced.

This location with you before or perhaps there are people you longed to share this special place with whom you have yet to experience this moment. So you invite them in and as if you are at a party in your honor. You enjoy feeling confident and feeling loved. Your generosity of spirit and sharing warms. The crowd like a late day Sun is sending out the vibrations you need to attract what you deserve honoring yourself. Honoring the beauty of your special place, honoring the memories of joy, you have carried with you the playful and carefree side of you. The red carpet that unrolls ahead that will guide you to more joyous and happy adventures to come. You have a lifetime to fill with more of these precious experiences, and with your community around you, I'll adorn in other costumes. That is jovial and vibrant and set to a theme that most inspires. You feel at peace you think stillness you feel plugged into the flow of your life's force. The vibrant beauty of your spirit and how lovely it is to be you how beautiful it is to be loved by all those who have been invited to share in the fun. So often, we may forget to prioritize joy. But right now, you're able to embrace it and feel fully and deeply carved within. You are a reminder to ignite fun and to revisit places that let you embrace the side of yourself in the future.

Because you can choose to be joyous and silly and have fun whenever you so desire, you may need a reminder as the sun sets upon the day in the setting of your favorite design and location. You may find the experience is fading away like a watercolor dream misty. Gray, the Technicolor fades, and you find yourself taking the glittering Rainbow Bridge between your waking and sleeping light. This bridge feels solid beneath your tired feet as you say goodbye to all those you invited along knowing. They will meet you in the dreams that come that you will be able to find respite and celebration tonight.

As you fall asleep, giving in to the darkness and the heaviness of your body. As you go deeper and deeper within as you go deeper and deeper down. I will count you down to a healing and restorative sleep to sleep that you have earned, let go, and finding peace. As you inhale and exhale, the words release me ten nine-eight seven-five-two-one binding bliss finding respite. Finding sleep, it's time to dream away a good night.

The Deep Dive

Take a moment to close your eyes. You can begin to relax in your way. You're out on this small boat at nighttime, and you can look around and notice the stars in the sky twinkling away, looking up and seeing the Milky Way stretching from one side of the horizon across the sky and down the other side. You can notice as you gaze up at the sky, different colors. The occasional plane that flies over and the sparkling sound of York meteorite that you see pass overhead. You can just relax on the boat as you're traveling to your dive site and as you relax on the ship while going to the dive site. You can notice the ship moving in the water, feeling the boat gently rocking up and down. As it moves through the waves and there's some movement even though the seas calm. As the night continues and you continue to go towards that dive site. So you can notice the moon rising on the horizon, seeing how there's bright white shimmering light on the water. As you gaze off, you notice that bright white shimmering light is dancing on the water's surface. You can see the waves moving and making light dance across the ocean, and you occasionally hear whales and dolphins breaching the surface. As they come up for air, take a breath blow out all their atmosphere, and dive back down again. The atmosphere is cooled and comfortable breathing that cool Aryan feels refreshing, so relaxing was like breathing in some healing.

When you breathe out, it's like breathing out any tension, you breathe in more healing and breathe out the stress. As you relax more profoundly and more comfortably and just enjoy the journey, almost like the boat moving on, the water reminds. You on some level of being rocked gently to sleep like a baby.

Something is calming and comfortable about this journey on this boat. You can hear the waves sloshing gently against the sides of the boat. Here the faint background chatter of the other divers among themselves. While you're just busy relaxing with your eyes closed now, just taking in some of that fresh sea air is just breathing that in and relaxing. Only allowing that relaxation to help your shoulders relax your neck muscles relax the muscles around your face. In your head, relax the muscles down through your back around your sides down your chest and down into your stomach relax. The muscles down way through your legs and your arms relax, resting on that boat having a sense of relaxation, just enjoying being in the moment not thinking about the past or worrying about the future being present at the moment thinking to yourself what a gift this moment is just enjoying being in the moment, Matt.

As the boat continues, you hear someone saying you're nearly at the dive site you've been looking forward to this dive for some time. As the moon has risen a bit higher, you notice how it lights up some clouds in the sky. How some of the clouds drift across the face of the moon, that's. Then the dive site they drop the anchor, and you can hear the chain unwinding the anchor drops more profound and deeper and deeper out of sight down into the ocean falling deeper and deeper. As the chain continues relaxing and when the chain finishes unwinding, you know that the anchor has reached the bottom. You go and get your diving gear on, and the other divers get their diving gear on. Then you put the face mask on you, hold the mouthpiece in your mouth, and do a couple of breaths. Just to test, it's all okay to check your equipment gives an okay signal sit on the edge of the boat. Then you allow yourself just to tip back into the water splashing into the water with your back and hearing. The sound of bubbles as you sink through the water and feel that weightlessness and instantly feel your breathing calming relaxing. As you start instinctively breathing with divers breathing, doing long full breaths from deep in your stomach breathing in and then breathing out.

Hearing the bubbles rise beside you and now and then as you move into the bubbles, you feel a tickling sensation from the bubbles on the side of your face. The water is a comfortable temperature; it's the kind of heat where almost feels like you're not even in water. All that nighttime, everything's crystal clear, and you've got your torch out, and you turn your light on. You wave the beam around, and you see the bottom when you see a shipwreck down there. You signal to the other divers to go ahead towards the sinking and with effortless movements of your feet. You feel propelled through the water go and deal even deeper into the darkness more profound and deeper toward that shipwreck. The boat above has some low noises coming from it, and the sound underwater is different from the sound at the surface. You can hear the wind. You can listen to sloshing and choppy water bouncing on the boat down here. It's just peace and calm like everything's running and a different speed more relaxed, giving you a sense of serenity as you start roaming around the shipwreck, having a sense of wonder of curiosity of intrigue. You see, the sinking has been here quite a while. They're ready many colonies of plants and fish and aquatic life growing and living in around the shipwreck that you swim inside the ship. You admire the wood, and you can hear the calming sound bubbles of in-breath out-breath. You travel deeper and deeper into this ancient shipwreck.

You realize this shipwreck is many hundreds of years old. You swim through this shipwreck, and you come out into what looks like a grand pool that was within the ship. You see, plates that looked like they could be cleaned up a bit and put into a cupboard or served up on tables. You see, sparkling cutlery that catches the light from your talk continues more in-depth into the ship. You discover different treasures in the ship you find glistening gold that looks as fresh and new today as when it landed on the bottom of the ocean gold coins with unrecognizable faces. You swim more profound and deeper into the ship before coming out of the other side of the boat right at the bottom of the ocean. While you just gaze around moving your legs gently to hover, keep yourself there you notice something that looks human-made under the sand on the seafloor. So you swim over, and you signal to some of the other divers to swim over as well, and you notice that it's a statue an ancient statue from an ancient civilization. It doesn't look familiar. You brush away a bit more of the sand; then you find that the statue is just part of something larger part of a whole community; it looks like there's a road.

Some statues and so you swim along this underwater road explore where it's going to go and keep an eye on your air levels. You've got plenty of time, and you can relax, and you swim along. The road seems to start heading down, and so you follow it deeper and deeper following it towards. Underwater Hill, only when you arrive at the hill, you shine the torch on it. The light seems to pick out some glistening stones, almost like someone's implanted diamond dust in the rocks. You run your hand along with that, and you swim around it and then find an entrance. This is an ancient pyramid, but for some reason is now deep under the sea, you've never heard of an ancient civilization in these parts. Where you're currently diving who you knew about was the shipwreck, you're going to dive down to see. You decide you want to explore the pyramid and swim into the tomb, swim through into the chambers. Then following the tunnels inside the pyramid, you find a tunnel heading up at a 45-degree angle. You swear that in that tunnel and see what looks like a door. You think there's no way you'd be able to move that door because it's mostly just a giant stone slab. But when you touch it, it's almost like you barely touched it.

Yet somehow it opened it went in, and then it slid along, and some of the water ran into the chamber, almost like sucking you up into that chamber. But it only filled the room a little way, so you opened that chamber without realizing that it wasn't flooded. You swam into the place thoroughly and understood that you could break the water's surface, and you don't know what the air will be like, but take your mask off to find out. You realize you're breathing air that hasn't been breathed in thousands of years. You shine your torch around the walls, glistening with gold with bright artwork and symbols. You feel a sense like somehow the artwork the experience you're having is teaching you something that this ancient civilization knew deep down and fundamentally. You see that at the far side of this chamber is another passage, and it's above the line where the water is flooded. So you climb out of the water, you walk across that bit of chamber and open the entrance to the passage. You start making a journey deeper and deeper into the pyramid. You don't yet know what you'll find. But you're curious how long this pyramid has been underwater for. If it's been underwater for a long time, it is doubtful to have been looted. And you nevermore know what you may find, and your footsteps echo.

As you walk down the corridor, you've taken off your flippers to help you walk better. You feel a sense of excitement, wonder, and curiosity and then find a - for the different artifacts made of different types of woods metals gold silver. You see, what looks a bit like an Egyptian sarcophagus only far more ancient, and you decide just to leave it. You don't need to disturb whoever's in there, but you look around the walls. You take in the symbols, and you realize that some of them aren't just symbols. It's only drawings like you would draw to artwork over critical events. You see animals on the walls drawn that you've never seen before, and you see Coastlines drawn on what looks like a map. Some of which you recognize, but it's not quite in the right place, and then you find some evidence that looks like. This is a different species of human the left Africa and evolved a whole civilization many thousands of years. Before I'm a sapiens left Africa and formed their culture. Something happened to this civilization and based on the fact that there's a pyramid and what it resembled the Egyptian pyramids that were far older. The main monuments and many other ancient civilizations pyramids and rituals. It seems like this civilization perhaps passed on summers messages, and then you think back to the stories. You'd heard about how the Egyptians used to talk about a traveler who arrived and gave them the knowledge of the gods to build pyramids.

Knowing what they need to do, there's an afterlife, and you now think that it seems those travelers may have been this ancient race of humans. You take your camera out of his underwater casing. You take a few photos before putting it back in its housing. You explore, get more around this pyramid, and you know you may never get a chance to come back here again. You finish up looking when you're ready to find your way back to where you came in and keep diving gear back on properly. Your face masks back on you, plop yourself down into the water and swim back out as the pyramid. You don't know whether anyone else will have decided to venture to the monument to look around it or inside. You start swimming back following that road back towards the shipwreck. As you swim, you can gaze up and notice how the moonlight flicks in glycerin, glistening and dancing in the water's surface, making shards of moonlight dance just under the surface. You can see shoals of fish swimming and dart around within those shards of light. Then you notice this dark shadow move across your field of vision up near the surface.

You realize it's a great white shark, and you're excited by this excited by the prospect of being in the water. So close to such a magnificent animal and so you relax on the bottom gazing up towards. The surface breathing calmly and softly watching the shark as it circles it swims along, so majestic can relax seeming to float so effortlessly. Then once the shark has swum around, you just watch as it swims off into the distance, then you head back along the edge of the boat back along the side of that ship underwater before starting to make your way up towards the surface. You know you're going to be taking a long while making your way up to the surface. You stop at regular intervals and hold your position to make sure you reach the surface safely. While you're holding a post, some dolphins come over, and one dolphin seems to hover itself just in front of your face. It seems to be penetrating you with clicks and whistles as if it's scanning you to figure out what kind of a person you are. Then it turns itself upside down about your waist level. You instinctively reach out and rub its belly, and it makes some clicks and whistles.

You interpreters it's enjoying itself, and it seems to be remaining in that position. So it looks comfortable to be having done what's happening. Then it turns back over again and swims around you, then it blows out a whistle and blows out a circular bubble. Another bubble expands and expands it swims and dives and splashes through that bubble coming up to the surface. Breaching the surface jumping cleared out of the water before gracefully dropping back into the water nose first again diving down to sea almost like once your approval, it's also trying to size you up swims around you. It rubs itself against you in the same way that a cat or a dog might rub itself against you. Then you get the okay you can rise a bit higher in the ocean. So you climb a bit higher, and the dolphin comes with you. The dolphin continues to splash around, you be playful around you, and after some time, you make it to the surface. While you're bobbing on the surface so that dolphin continues to swim around, you want to play with you. This wouldn't go past you; it seems to encourage you to hold on to his fin. So you do hold on to his paddle and relax and enjoy the fast ride around in a circle before it decides.

When to make you let go and while you're bobbing on the surface, you hear the loud sound of a whale blowing out its air. You see that a sperm whale that's just surfaced quite near to you, and you're in awe of that whale's size. It doesn't seem to register that you're there doesn't seem to care that you're there. It just breaches. The surface lets out its air before facing back down again and diving way down into the depths thousands of meters lower. You just being, and you just barb on the surface for a while. You wait for the boat just to get a bit closer. So you can climb up and get out when you're out of the water you get out of your scuba gear you take some time to sit down just gaze out over the sea. Just enjoy watching that dolphin the other dolphins play in the sea visible. In the moonlight jumping high out the water and landing on their backs, jumping out the pool is doing flips and going those first back into the water without hardly a splash.

Then you find by watching nature by watching these dolphins by watching whales. When they breach and let their air out and dive deep again, you see this so relaxing and thoughts become relaxing, and thoughts relax you no, it's a long journey back to the shore. She finds a small bed on the boat to settle down and while you settle down and that little bed. So your mind wanders two exciting stories, almost like long-lost memories of ancient lives of this ancient civilization. You fall asleep imagining the ancient civilization imagining its culture what it looks like how they dressed where they lived trying to piece together. This information from the photos you took and what you learned and realizing the importance of your breathing and control over that calm, relaxed breathing. The critical component of diving successfully. So you mentally her has new drift off to sleep. Imagine different scenarios in different settings and wonder what the future will hold for your discoveries—looking forward to coming out again to go on that dive.

The Lost Pyramid

Take a moment to close your eyes. You can begin to relax in your way. While you drift and start to dream so I'll talk to you in the background, speak to you about the discovery of a Lost pyramid. You can have a sense of being in Egypt and gently rowing down the Nile. The sound of the oar is you push the water back on one side of your bones, lift the or over the boat and push the water back on the other side of your boat. The sound of the water sloshing being pushed back the sound of water dripping back into the water. As the August lifted out from one side and lowered into the other hand and that pressure and that feeling of the oar. As it passes through the water and propels you comfortably further along the river. As you continue to grow along the river, you can feel the sun's warmth on your face. Perhaps you've got a hat on to shield you a little from some of that Sun as you continue to roll along the river. You can hear sounds around you sounds of people on the shore sounds of music sounds of the hustle and bustle sounds of birds. In the sky, some darting around some is just hovering there, occasionally casting shadows on the ground from the water. You can be aware of the different colors and shades that you can see the different textures. As you can see, new rowing down the river and occasionally you can notice how the river just gets slightly choppy.

The boat just Bob's on that choppy water before straightening and continuing smoothly along the river. You're looking for something that stands out. You've heard rumors that somewhere along the river. You used to be a pyramid a long-lost pyramid, and you don't know really what you're looking for, just something that stands out something slightly unusual. Something that doesn't seem natural and as you continue along the river. So you begin to move further away from the built-up areas around the riverbank. The sounds around you start to quiet them down, begin to relax, and everything begins to feel more peaceful karma. As you continue and then some way down the river, you pull over to the shore, you row the boat just gently slightly up onto the beach. I'm out the front of the boat and have that sense of pulling the boat up the shore somewhat out of the water, noticing ours. You pull it out of the water your feet give in the soil and that gravelly sound of pulling the boat up onto the shore. You can feel a slight breeze from time to time on your face, and perhaps your face starts to get warm. Maybe your cheeks begin to fill warm as you relax, and you take a moment to be observant of looking around you very slowly.

Move your head around, take in what you can see calmly looking around, just looking for something that stands out of the ordinary. And you decide to do something you've never tried before, and you don't think anyone else has. You get your camera out you set your camera so that it's cut high contrast, and you look through your camera. You look for areas that seem to stand out against the background. You notice that some vegetation just looks slightly different to the rest seems a little peculiar. It appears to be formed in a somewhat more straight-line than you'd expect by chance or naturally in this area. You can take over to walk over to that area, and as you do, you notice long rough grass that's standing slightly taller in two straight lines from the lines. Just over a body's width apart better foot and a half apart perhaps two feet, and you walk between the lines. As you walk between the lines of grass there, you notice how the soil feels different; this seems to be spring air appears to have a bit more give not entirely. As far as the soil just outside of those two lines.

90

So you get a shovel from your bag on your back, and you start digging. After digging for a little while, you notice that there seems to be a staircase going under the ground. So you dig and see the stairs new hit a step and have that clunk of hitting the stage. So you scrape that step clean, and then you dig, dig, and hit another level. So you scrape that step clean, then move forward a bit and dig and dig you catch another action. So you scrape that step clean and then move forward a bit further, and you dig, and you dig and keep repeating this going deeper and deeper. You notice as you go more profound than the Sun can't quite reach you, so you suddenly feel more relaxed even though you're digging. So you keep digging until you reach a point where there seems to be a floor at the bottom of this staircase. So you dig forward along the floor, and you dig up. And you start digging under the ground, and you discover that you're in a slight tunnel.

As you dig into this tunnel, so you start feeling a little excitement, wondering what it is you've discovered and where you are, and you reach a door a stone slab. So you scrape the stone slab clean clear all the mud from the stone slab. You notice that this stone slab has been placed here in a particular way. There are two bits of wood in the bottom corners of the stone slab, and you pull on those bits of wood. Suddenly the stone slab rolls back towards you, and you jump back out the way, jumping back onto the steps. The piece hits the steps and stops with a thud, and you climb up over that slab go back to the door. There's a certain rosamma like the air hasn't been breathed for years, and you wonder if this is the lost tomb' you're looking for, you know it's a tomb that's been lost. So you get your torch and flick your light on beginning to walk into the corridor. That suddenly opens up before you, and it's pitch-black apart from what your view is lighting.

You notice hieroglyphs around the walls, and you take a few photos of some of those hieroglyphs. You hear the echoing footsteps that you accept and from the sound of the steps. The echo you can listen to, you can deduce that this is a very long tunnel, and the air is still. After perhaps five or ten minutes of walking, the tube begins to veer upwards. So you follow the tunnel upwards, then it turns around to the right. So you follow it round to the right, and then there's a vertical shaft. So although it's quite a struggle, you climb up that vertical shaft putting your back against one wall flicking your feet up on to the other wall, and walking up the vertical axis. Then your muscles constrained and take your weight, and it can be a huge struggle to get up that vertical shaft when you reach the top. You scramble up onto the surface you roll onto your back and relax and just do some deep breaths to let that tension go to make your muscles relax. And then, after your muscles relax and you feel ready to carry on your journey. You pick your torch up and shine it around, and you notice this is a vast chamber. In the distance as you waved your torch around something listened. So you decide to head towards whatever it was the glistened.

Now the echoes sound like you're in a cathedral or a church each footstep that you take echoes like you're in some kind of a vast area. You shine your torch up, and yet the light just gets lost in the darkness. When you arrive at that thing that reflected and glistened, you discover it's a hieroglyphic symbol printed in gold like someone had poured gold onto the wall. While it was drying stamped in that gold with a hieroglyph for a pharaoh, you discover that this is the place you were looking for because that symbol is for Pharaoh from an age before Pharaohs from a lost ancient civilization that gave rise to the known Pharaohs. Then you can notice your heart speeding up a little at the excitement of what you've discovered as you focus on this and wonder with curiosity what's behind that door. You know you should wait and go and get a team to do a proper investigation. But you can't expect it. This was a lifelong obsession discovering this tomb. Now you're here, and it looks like no one has ever been in here since it was sealed your assumption at this point is that it can't have been looted. Because where else that gold seal would have been stolen and say use your shovel to prise the door open and some of the air from inside the chamber.

You're in getting sucked into the room you've just exposed almost as you've just opened an airlock. You think about how you're breathing air that's been in this tomb since it was sealed thousands of years ago. Then you notice the other side of the door are some unlit torches. So you get your lighter out, and you light the torches as soon as you light the torches. The entire room lights up and reflects you notice as a chamber made of gold the floor the ceiling. The walls are all gold bright and glistening with wooden and golden artifacts golden sarcophagus, and much of this you notice is unmovable, it's so reliable. So massive and yet so exciting, you're the first to see this in thousands of years. At the back of the tomb, there's a painting, and it doesn't look like the Egyptian art on the walls. That person is familiar with it; it looks like a painting that could have been done. During the Renaissance, almost like a lifelike depiction and you can notice in that depiction in that large painting, the individual through the portrait is of who's most likely the person in the sarcophagus. You can see in the background painting what the place looked like back then noticing what people were doing a picture of people milling around the art of people going to markets painting people.

Just going about their daily lives, and you can notice that be fascinated that only that one picture gives a snapshot of what everything looked like back. Then almost as if when this was drawn that Pharaoh had to sit incredibly still on a veranda in an elevated location. While the artist drew and painted, then sat there and the scene in the background of the ancient lost city of people going about their daily business of healthy life. The kind of thing that's so easy to get lost with history. As you walk around the painting and you look closely at the different aspects. In that painting, so you notice a slight breeze coming from behind the picture. So you take a moment to shift that painting and just slide that painting over a little. You realize there's a tunnel behind the art. You follow that tunnel. Then you find more torches to light, and you light those torches and as you go around burning all the flames. So you find that you've just discovered a vast chamber containing an entire army of chariots soldiers in army uniform. The horse is ideally in rows and the middle of this chamber. You find out a giant golden pool full of mercury, and then, the light glistens and sparkles and bounces off precious stones and gems throughout this chamber.

You notice a giant golden disc being lit up by the light and partially obscuring it up on one of the walls. You notice a perfectly polished giant black disc, and coming off the black drive, you see what looks like the head of a snake tailing off. As you follow it into a body of a snake and you realize that this is a special place and particular symbology of the worship of the Sun. The way every night darkness swallowed the Sun and every morning, the Sun won the battle and rose again like a phoenix rising from the ashes. You take some time to take photos of different things. In the air sitting quietly, just enjoying peace enjoying the atmosphere enjoying knowing that you're the first person in perhaps 10,000 or more years to have discovered. This place to found the tomb of this long-lost Pharaoh that goes way back to an ancient civilization. Before the familiar Egyptian civilizations, you take some time to try and work out your bearings. You're aware this is a vast location, and you realize how far you've dug how far you walked down the tunnel. That this must be inside the nearby mountain that perhaps. Now, as you think about it isn't a mountain.

It's an ancient pyramid that's been covered over perhaps intentionally to hide it. That's been lost through history because you're aware from the outside that mountain that huge hill just looks like a weathered hill. So you can take some time of peace here, taking all the time to explore to discover more. While you do, you notice something seeming to throw up with light, and you go over to it. You rest the palm of your hand on it, and as you relax, the palm of your hand on it. So you suddenly seem to does that pew into the past into some kind of vision of the past like a virtual reality machine that seems to zap you back into the past. Almost like an old virtual reality machine to teach future generations about history and technology. They had zapped you into the past, and as you fall asleep. Now, so you can dream that past finding yourself looking through your eyes hearing through your ears feel what you feel in the past as if you were in the background of that old painting in a busy marketplace in ancient Egypt, thousands and thousands of years ago. As you drift comfortably asleep.

The Monarch Butterfly

Get ready to fall asleep tonight with a guided sleep meditation and story that will help you relax in sweet surrender. At the end of summer has marveled humanity for centuries as these delicate yet Hardy creatures letter their way from the northeastern seaboard of the United States - as far as Mexico to seek respite from the cold winter. In this story, you will be able to travel along on this great migration before falling into a deep and healing sleep as you get cozy and dive into your sleep ritual. You may let go of your day and find your chest, heart, and lungs feeling lighter, imagining the lightness of being that a monarch butterfly enjoys throughout its life. As you sink into your bed and let your eyelids flutter closed before resting heavily upon your tired eyes inhaling and exhaling. As you tune into your breath, slowing it down, and as you inhale, you visualize the words; I am on the backs of your eyelids and exhale as the words light and carefree appear like a cursive neon-lit sign and inhaling. You see the words I am and then exhale to understand the terms letting go. This deep breath creates a rhythm, a soft and comfortable tempo that matches the gentle flutter of monarch butterflies' velvety wings. She glides above the golden sands of a barrier island at summers.

She is your guide on this journey, and you deeply trust her as young as she may be. She has been born with a roadmap and plans, just like you have been born with a roadmap and strong pull of intuition to guide you towards experiences. And people are meant to be a part of the tapestry of your life. This glorious monarch lands of harm the wet sand that now glitters like tiny golden topaz and diamond gemstones her feet. Taste the briny waters that

I've washed the shore and naturally say and protected from the seagulls. Now feasting as her glorious black dots and stripes, orange and white pattern indicates to pray that she is poisonous to consume. So she is free to explore fearlessly and without a care and just as you may recall times in your life. When the Sun's warmth gave you energy and awakened you in a new day, the monarch butterfly no absorbs heat from the Sun that rises over the horizon. So she may begin her great migration southerly to escape the harshness of winter. You can experience all the sensations in this beautiful and safe mental state between your waking and sleeping life. This butterfly feels the comforting warmth from the Sun and the intuitive poll and understanding of where she must go, and you relish in her certainty. How she can commit to part of the journey without concern about the final destination, the migration is all about answering the call one day at a time for this monarch one flap of her papery wings.

At a time and just like you have transformed into different physical versions of yourself, the metamorphosis of this monarch from caterpillar to butterfly gives you a sense of relief, and growth and transformation are not just a conscious decision. They are often a requirement to serve me, and the greatest of growth may flow if you listen and tune in to your intuition and needs. Gently and calmly accepting this is part of being alive, and as the Sun begins to rise higher above the horizon and glittering sapphire sea illuminating the sky. The temperature starts to increase the air becomes misty from a haze of silvery-blue morning fog that coats. The warm golden sands the ocean is at its warmest temperature after months of intense July and August heat. Long days of sunlight have transformed it into a heated saltwater bath. The monarch takes one last solo pass across the shoreline. The same shore she may return to come springtime, she is full of energy and life vivacity. As brilliant as the vibrancy of her velvety orange hue wings. She flutters inland towards a pine home that has been faded by the salty air. Lands upon potted zinnias in shades of fuchsia and purple and marigold yellow. She was sitting in the nectar that coats our black feet with its intoxicating fragrance filling up.

Other monarchs join her, also getting in their nourishment before the great flight southward begins. Then just like the streams of an orchestra that is warming up for a performance, the first of the swarm of butterflies begin to take to the cerulean blue skies going higher and higher. You can feel the splendor of what this is like this easy ascent towards. The sky fluttering up and up as a wind assists their plight like a summers wind hitting the sails of a boat out at sea-salty air has the slightest net. The cut through the otherwise warm morning's temperature is a gentle battle between the heat of the Sun and autumns chill. But for now, the warmth winds out during daylight hours, and the monarch butterflies inherently understand this and use this particular time to begin their epic journey. You feel how freeing it has the support of the breeze beneath your monarch guides wings that seamlessly Blyde forward, able to travel up to 100 miles or 160 kilometers. A day relies on the gold and sun to activate and support their journey; the monarchs travel above the visto of lush emerald green marshes. Waterways along the Seaboard and human-made homes that scatter the landscape below the trees are beginning to change colors.

While predominantly a verdant green, it is as if the forest below is speckled with hops of gold, magenta, and orange leg, a mystical speckled egg from a distance. It is so natural and comfortable to appreciate the splendor of the planet below, and you take it in the brightness of the experience. The wonder of being such a small yet resilient life-form a flock of seagulls flies in the opposite direction sharing the open skies that are so vast. Yet offer a sense of community for all air-bound creatures. They have been gifted with skills that take them away from the land-bound and water-bound species below and right. Now relish their ability to soar the landscape below becomes meditative a continual kaleidoscope of life basking in the afternoon's Sun. You think back to all the times in your life as a child or even in the dreamscapes of your sleeping life where you imagined what it would feel like to fly how wondrous. It would be to escape the strong pull of gravity and to look at the planet from a new vantage point as you inhale and exhale looking through the eyes and living the experience of this monarch butterfly. You intake all the sensations of this journey what it is like to be. So light and feathery and yet so durable and determined with a set direction and end goal to be so beautiful and vibrant with velvety soft wings. That seems so fragile and again can endure four months of light during migration to appear.

So captivating and delicate and yet simultaneously convey a sense of danger to all potential predators how perfect it is to be a butterfly. You relish in this protection, and as you go deeper and deeper within, you realize that you, too, are part of perfection. You are here to learn to grow and to transform, and you are doing that every single new day you're opening yourself to new experiences. You're tending to your basic needs for relaxation and respite at the end of the day. You may take this moment to celebrate you to celebrate the spectacular moment in time that you had this shift. You answered this call to work towards being your best self to aligning yourself with the greater good for you to listening to that intuitive voice that begins. As a whisper and can become as loud as necessary until you hear your inner voice. On this light, this intuitive journey of the monarch butterflies you vow to go deeper and deeper within does their ender and listen to your truth. To the guidance that the universe is always offering to you like two dials in your heart center reminiscent of an old radio dial, you may tune in to the right frequency and with the other dial. You may tune up the volume until you hear what needs to be heard, and you're doing so very well feeling so relaxed.

The day is beginning to fade into the night, and the kaleidoscope of monarch butterflies are slowing down and light during the hottest point of the day the Monarchs were able to ascend. As high as 10,000 feet or 3,000 meters above the Earth's surface as the temperature drops. The Sun lowers beyond the horizon the last of the liquid orange waves of light spanning the landscape in deciduous and evergreen trees. Below the Monarchs begin to lower intuitively aware they may drop out of the sky if the temperature decreases to significantly gently gliding down beneath the shadows of the trees flattering as autumn leaves on a night wind. The air clean and Kris the aromas of the forest floor and behind trees swirling up through the spaces between feathery branches becoming more fragrant. The further and further down towards the ground, the Monarchs have loved your monarch guide leads. The swarm of butterflies settling among the damp branches of a pine tree all settling Emirati branches their feet is taking in the sticky pine pitch's aroma. You feel what it's like to nestle among the owls and squirrels and deer and birds and rabbits that I've all gotten cozy for the night. I ready to surrender to their tiredness. It is the completion of another day and for the monarch butterflies. This journey will continue for months, with each day finding them.

A first-time glimpse has new parts of the continent, and each night will bring a comfortable retreat or respite. You may think of your life in the same way no day is ever the same, even if you are doing the same things. You are different each day the circumstances change. So many new things await being discovered by you. Each night welcomes you like a gentle hug and unique sanctuary offering you sleep—an escape from your toils and challenges of each day. In the months that come like centuries ago, people will await the arrival of the swarms of butterflies seeking escape from the cold their iconic wings, bringing them to a new place. How spreading beauty across the land monarch butterflies serving as nature's most beautiful hand-painted canvas. Just as they are awaited, there are people in the future that welcome and await you as you grow and transform on your journey. You are free to explore the intuitive urges and a divine inner voice within us all and with a peaceful hum of the forest. The sacred sound of crickets and a babbling brook you are welcome to find piece and rasp it to find sleep to get cozy and relaxed to get all the rest. It would be best if you continued to grow and transform - let the blank canvas of your dreams awaits you tonight to be painted with the same beauty that accompanies the journey. You have earned this moment you deserve this. You're worthy of the peace and stillness that accompanies you as you are ready to let go and slip into a dream world of bliss. I am going to count you down to this place for healing sleep feeling so heavy and relaxed ten nine eight seven six by three to one finding rest finding stillness. Finding sleep, it's time to dream away goodnight.

You're Okay, And It's All Good

While asleep easily and quickly with our guidance. Sleep meditation, you may find comfort and safety as these feelings wrap around you like a childhood blanket and allow you to trust in yourself. In your life, at times in life, there may win out over love and joy like a switch that turns on a light. So - may you turn on an internal switch to illuminate the dark corners. Where anxiety and fear and self-doubt. May lurk it may not be easy, but it is most certainly possible I would like to welcome you to Michelle Sanctuary. You are listening to healing sleep meditation. Your okay, and it's all good. This talk down will help you make peace with your path with all the challenges of the past.

All that may be currently troubling you right now will allow you to relax and unwind deeply. Let it all go right now; let it all just go you don't need it. You never did. You don't need to hold on to anything. You may even visualize the gates of a levee opening and releasing a reservoir of water into the sea, allowing all your thoughts and concerns to flow out and merge with something vast and expansive. Suddenly your problems seem quite small it is no longer your responsibility to keep all of this is because you are okay. It is all good, yes, you are okay, and it is all good and perhaps. You may remember a time in your life when you are scared are not feeling well. We're comforted by someone who loves you very much in the safety of an embrace are imagining the fingers of a loved one.

One gently brushing your hair away from your face; you may hear this kind whisper. How true-time proved it to be right it's going to be okay you are going to be okay. Nothing stays. The same forever, this too shall pass you are okay. You are going to be just fine. Maybe you don't have it all figured out. Perhaps you don't know much about it. This adulting business and you're tired of trying to figure it all out. But you need not worry or figure it out tonight. You know you don't even need to completely figure it out in this lifetime at all because no one has completely figured out life. As it unfolds is a continuous series of lessons an education that you may learn from, and if you don't learn the first time, you will surely be given time. Time again, one experience after the next to be given another chance to try and learn the lesson time to figure it out. There is plenty of time ahead; there is not a deadline for you that pressure may just put more anxiety into a toolbox that should be full of tools. An arsenal of all your strengths and wisdom intuition and creativity should be allowed every inch of space; those worries are not worth space.

They try to take up, and you deserve to have love and self-acceptance and nurture yourself and to feel nurtured by those around you. Because you are doing just fine, you are okay. It is all good, and your mind and emotions indicate how you feel and what stories you may tell yourself about yourself. You may change the story; you may readjust the way you process and think about things. You may make a choice right now to feel good to feel safe to say to yourself I am okay. And I am doing the best that I can do, given all the experiences. I have been given I am trying I can fall and get back up again. I can listen to my inner voice and guidance. I can acknowledge that deep down, I have my inner compass to guide me. I can trust that I can find stillness deep within I can seek a sanctuary to heal my wounds. To get healthy again so I can go into the world and thrive, I am doing the best I can for myself and for forgiving others. Because forgiveness is the best gift, I may give to myself and to those who have hurt or disappointed me or just let me down. Because it is all part of the human experience, you are only human. So is everyone else around you, and it's okay, and it's all good, our life is all about choices. We are the ones in charge of these choices. So right now, in your sanctuary and within the safety of your mind. You may go deeper and deeper within and go to the steady warm flow of peace that comes.

You may even let these words drift across the movie screens on the backs of your dark closed eyelids as you sudden. These mantras and messages way up here in any style font let any way on the screen that you desire I choose to forgive. I want to let go. I want to recognize what is in my control and to surrender what is not I want to believe that. I came to this life to learn and that the hardships I experienced are meant to bring me closer to what I need and desire. I choose to trust I want to honor me. As used to let go of pride and my ego for the sake of love and happiness. I want to listen to my intuition. I want to listen to everything and everyone around me. So I may learn and grow I want empathy I'd want to recognize my strengths and embrace it. I want to be me. I choose to let myself shine; I choose to love myself. I choose to be brave; it's used to acknowledge that everyone around me has been afraid of dealing with their limitations. Their fears, I choose to recognize my fear. So I may overcome it, I choose to deal with myself I choose to honor my past but embrace the present. I choose to connect with others. I choose to connect with my presence so that I may be led to the future. I most desire I decide to accept that I have a finite time that is precious in this life to do all the things. I need to do and to say all the things I need to say I choose to try; I choose to believe I choose to be okay with everything right now.

I choose to feel okay because I am okay, and it is all good. As you feel your body relaxing, your muscles are melting. All that you have been carrying with you all that as a wage you down may be released from your body. You no longer need to take all that weight. Maybe right now, you are just becoming aware of all that has been haunting you and holding you back. You may let go of these blocks to your creativity into your journey because you are okay. It is all good. You may not know your direction; you may not know what you want, but it is okay. If this is so, then your current life's purpose is to discover what you want, and if or when you find out this, you are ready and able to go. After what you wish to because it is yours and you can do this, you've got this. You are doing just fine. Even when you feel like you are not enough, you may trust me. As I say this, you are enough; you are everything you need to be every step has gotten to where you are right now. So you need not live and regret it because you are here directly. Right here on the right path, and you know this because you took the time to find a sanctuary and to connect, you took the time to come here.

Just accept that everything is okay. Everything is just as it should be right now, and you are doing all you need to be doing just breathing in and out. Because one conscious breath is a meditation, you're able to take another conscious breath inhaling and believing. In the mystical powers, the cause synchronicity that caused things to come together at the right time. In the right place that brings you to a state of wonder and faith. Right now, the trust begins with you was believing in yourself; it just takes the tiniest spark of belief right now to ignite a fire that will burn within you. Because it is all right thinking about how many problems you have already solved in this life, in this year, in this month in the week and even today, how many things you had overcome even when you did not want to be faced with them. Every time you overcame, you instill this deep memory that you can do this that you have already done hard things. Save prevailed. You're still here in any fears you may have about the end of life. May drift away because all you need to do is live each day to the fullest to make the most out of every moment. Every connection with those that you love that you may allow in new influences.

People that foster your growth and believe in you realize this right now say to yourself I am okay, I will be okay.

It is all good, and I am right, and this is good, and everything will be okay, and being alright does not mean perfect it. It does not mean things are how you want them to be all the time. It does not mean that everything is figured out that you have mastered the art of being an adult. But you've figured out everything about life, maybe you know even less now. Then you thought you knew before, and that is okay because being okay is a choice of acceptance and surrender. Being okay means, you are choosing your happiness and ease of being and balanced mind over unmet expectations and disappointment. We are all disappointed at times, and that is okay disappointment serve as an opportunity to tune you into what you want to light a fire in your heart to motivate. You to empower you to be brave enough to say perhaps at first in the chambers of your mind. Later to the world beyond you, I want this; I need this; I can no longer be afraid. I choose to do what it takes to get what I need and desire. May be right, we lose things a little bit at a time because it is all good. You may realize how much better it feels to just surrender like a sea turtle riding the waves of a gentle turquoise sea you too may ride along. Let go doing fine, recognizing what is in your control and what is not. You can control your feelings. You can manage your thoughts; you can control what choices you make; you can control how you express what you need and desire. You're very good at doing this.

You may be brave. You may accept that your feelings matter your thoughts matter. It's okay to have opinions that sometimes are intense. But sometimes, don't feel right. You are learning to embrace and acknowledge what they are. You are choosing to shine a light on what can be healed. Rather than burying it deep within and those voices that you sometimes hear, perhaps those who have influenced you caused you to have doubts within yourself. They may be silenced; maybe it is your voice creating chatter a causes anxiety and self-doubt that may now be released these voices. Never felt good anyway, so I hold on to them just as you would turn a radio dial when a song comes on that you do not enjoy. So - may you now change the thoughts in your mind surrender and drift towards. And all the things that make you feel good about yourself to think about everything that you love most about being you about something. You have done for others that make you feel good about the love you have been able to think about the bonds. You have formed in your life, reflecting on the chances. You have been given the times you have listened to your intuition and indeed allowed stillness to grant you the insight to guide your life, trusting that this voice is always.

There the useful inner guide that is you that has always been you the part of you that has existed throughout your entire life. You may find that voice growing louder, and like a watercolor painting left out in gentle spring rain, these thoughts become like watercolors that melt into your dreaming life. So you may continue to dream tonight and have guidance that will allow you to wake up feeling motivated and inspired. Because it's okay, you are okay and will be alright tomorrow and the days that come ahead. It is all good and feeling this lightness of being like a kite sailing across a clear sky. You are now free to cross the unique bridge into your dreaming life. This is a sacred time that comes at least once a day wheN you drift and surrender to the deep sleep and healing and empowering dreams that await you. You may go across this bridge, letting yourself float through the misty air. In the most ethereal of transitions going deeper and deeper down towards sleep towards dreams that show the acceptance. You have of being okay a feeling good about where you are with who you are because you are okay. It is all good, and I am going to count you down towards a restorative night of sleep that you have earned. So rightfully deserve where you may take in the lessons of the day. Explore the possibilities for two more lettings go of my voice letting go of your waking life 10 9 8 7 6 5 4 3 2 1 finding bliss finding healing finding peace finding out that it's all right it's time to dream away the excellent night.

Time Waits for No Man

Just allow your eyes to close and with your eyes closed. You can begin to drift comfortably asleep as you drift comfortably asleep. I don't know whether you'll fall asleep faster. You fall asleep; I'm just going to tell you a story. This person finds herself walking through a strange land, and she gazes out over that land. As she's walking along and she can see floating land. In the sky, she can see trees on that floating land mountains on the free land. She can see some of the open lands have waterfalls falling from that land down to the land below. She can notice that floating land appears to be tethered to other floating lands, almost like a matrix of floating lands. In the sky with huge tethers between each bit of land and then there are points where there are fasteners down to the ground. The brakes don't appear to be human-made. They seem to somehow it is part of the environment. She'd heard that in this land, there was the particular magnetic rock that there were areas where the magnetic stone would repel itself from the opposing magnetic force of other rock. So these floating areas were floating on a cushion of magnetism. She gazed out as far as the eye could see she could see the gaps in the ground. Where those areas had floated up into the sky, and she didn't know the cause of this land. In this way, she could see legs and the way the sun glistened on the Lake's surface.

She could see vast forests of tall trees with ink the occasional even more towering tree poking out the top some areas where there was mist across the top of the woods. She could notice the color of the sky clouds birds flying high. She gazed out across this land, and she'd never been here before he was on a journey. She had to find somebody she didn't know what that person would be like. But she knew she would know when she had seen them, so she walked down the hillside walked down into the forest started pushing through the woods. She clear-- the sounds in the different forest animals sounds of birds sounds of each footstep. She took as she pushed on through the woods then while she pushed through the woods. She wondered who this person would be. She was just told it's ahead west. She wasn't told how far or when she would meet that person, it's only known that she would recognize them and know that she's found them. She was told that they would happily talk to her and be very charming. She had something important she needed to learn from them. So she continued to push her way through the forest and as she pushed through the woods. She wondered about how she was making sure she could stay heading west.

She found that so much easier when she was out in a clearing where she could see the sky and be aware of her surroundings. After some time, she managed to clear the forest and reach a lake. She created herself a raft and then started paddling across the Lake on that round hear. The sound of the oar in the water she pushed forward the sound of the float moving through the water would smell the freshwater air. Notice the subtle missed the hovered just above the water's surface. So she rode across that Lake, and at the far side of the Lake, she dragged a makeshift craft up onto the shore covered. It over with some giant leaves in case she needed it and want anyone to take it. Then she carried on her journey west, and she came to a mountain and started climbing that mountain. As she rose, so trees thinned out till eventually, she was above the trees. She continued climbing and then she reached some snowy area. She kept climbing higher, and she and I jumped up and over the mountain range.

As she was on the other side of the mountain range. So she saw a dragon in the distance circling round above some forest, and looking around, she saw a bird of prey in another direction flocks of birds flying in formations. Sometimes birds launching themselves from the forest before landing elsewhere, she was aware of how much life was going on here just going about its. Everyday business while she was on this quest to find this wise person. She started down the mountain found it much more comfortable going down the hill. Then going up and as she was going down the hill. She noticed that there was running water down this side, flowing from the mountain. She started following that newly forming River, which gradually turned into more of a torrent of water and waterfalls. Then at the foot of the hill as the ground started leveling out, so the rain started slowing. The river started widening, and she felt it would be easier to follow the river's side. Then to have to keep pushing forward through the jungle. So she followed this river and after some time following this river she saw an ornate bridge and either side of that bridge was a road.

This Road looked like it had been well kept and so it must be an essential road leading somewhere. So she went to that bridge, and she saw that there was a man with a cane sitting on the deck. Just using the rod to prop himself up, and she greeted herself to him, and he greeted her back. Then he started talking to her in his charming and pleasant conversation. She wondered if this was the wise man she said that she was on a mission. She had to find something of importance, but she didn't know what but she was told that the wise man would know it's just head west. Until you see him. He said he'd been sat here waiting to be found, and she asked what you mean you've been sat here waiting to be discovered are you lost. He said that he's in precisely the right place for this moment if she asked him how can you be wanting to be found or needing to be found. If you're not lost, why don't you just go somewhere? He said he is somewhere, he said. He's in the middle of somewhere. He'd rather be somewhere than nowhere, and she asked him, but if you are somewhere. You're waiting to be found how did you know to expect to be seen how did you know someone was looking for you.

He said somebody is always looking and nobody finds anyone the only person that can find anyone is somebody who's searching. She discovered that his conversation was going through her head in some way. She didn't fully understand it at the moment. But it was so unusual she assumed this must be the wise man he then said her time stand still for no man. She thought that was a strange thing to say of course time doesn't stand still you told her. She's looking for time and when she's found the time she will have seen what she's searching for and she didn't understand. And she asked how do I find the time I don't have much time for this. I'm looking for something, and I don't even know what, and he explained that you do know what because I've told you you just have to take the time you need to discover it for yourself. He explained that all roads come to an end. So she has to decide which Road she wants to follow to that end. She asked, but one Road is probably the wrong Road, and the other Road is perhaps right. How do I know which Road to choose and he said you're right one Road is probably the wrong Road in the Road that's left is right? She thought to herself, how this doesn't help at all. She's no more transparent as to what Road to follow. He told her you to have all the answers. You just need to trust yourself and know that you know all the answers even if you don't know you know them. She thought to herself, and this man is of no help. She thought to herself that she's just going to wander down one of the roads. When she meets someone else, she'll ask them maybe they can speak more sense.

Maybe this isn't the wise person, so she got up and left - let's follow the left Road. She started thinking about the interaction started trying to process what he might have meant. The Road followed around along near the river and as she observed that Road. She allowed herself to get lost in thought. She found trains of thought stretching from one thing to another as she continued to walk as she tried to process and make sense of what the man had said. As she followed that Road, she could see across the river to the other Road. You could see that both roads look like they'll go in the same way just both on different sides. After many hours of walking, it was starting to get dark, and she'd crossed mountain she'd walked miles. She felt she needs asleep, so she set up camp lit a fire had something to eat took some time to meditate to drift off in her mind. In her thoughts to process her experiences. While she gazed at the flickering flames of the fire, she was aware of the blast dancing around, creating dance lights and shadows. In the night, the sound of the water in the background the sights of stars. In the sky, the sound of rustling leaves as the wind blew breeze as she then settled down and drifted comfortably asleep. As she drifted pleasantly asleep, so she started to dream.

While she dreamt, she replayed what that man had said only the man didn't look like the man in her dream. He didn't quite tell what he said, but she knew this was a representation of what she could learn from. She imagined herself picking up a mirror, a handheld mirror and holding it out in front of her, and looking at herself in that mirror. Then suddenly being propelled faster and faster through space getting quicker and quicker and quicker. She is noticing everything around her slowing down to the point where everything around her almost grinds to a halt. Whereas going so slow is practically invisible and she looks to the left, and she looks to the right. She looks up and looks down; she looks around her. Notices out everything it's almost ground to a halt, and she looks forward again. Notes that she can see her head-turning in the mirror and everything in the mirror is happening in real-time. Yet everything around her has slowed right down, and she knows somehow this is all connected. Yet she doesn't know how and she has this feeling like the sun's rising feeling of warmth on her face. She gradually opens her eyes holding on to this dream, and while she holds on to the idea. She continues her journey, and as she continues her journey, she notices that the Road on the other side of the river.

Suddenly comes to an abrupt halt as it drops steeply into a gap left by one of the floating islands. In the sky and yet the Road, she's on just misses the edge of that gap. She notices how that River abruptly becomes a waterfall pouring down into that gap she looks up at that floating island. She looks down into the difference she looks over at that other Road and realizes. If she'd been following that Road, it would have been a road to nowhere, and she'd have to turn around and walk back again. If she just followed the river, she'd have to have tried to steer to the shore. Before the river turned into that waterfall, she continued walking along the road, looking down into the gap and looking up at the island, walking around that gap. Until she'd passed the difference and carried on walking, she realized that perhaps that wise man was wise in the first place. Because what he had said was correct, it said the path that's left is right, and she got up and went following the left part. She did it without any thought at all. She just decided to get up and decided just to walk along that path. She didn't realize that she just did as he had said. It just happened instinctively and automatically. After some time further of walking along this path, she saw a palace the palace that no one lived in any longer. Yet it looked like everyone had left just a day ago despite no one living here for hundreds of years.

She walked into the palace grounds walked through those palace grounds passed ideally kept grounds of plants flowers shrubs as she entered the palace so she could hear a ticking clock, and she walked instinctively towards. The sound of that ticking clock somehow she felt was what she was after that she needed to find that ticking clock. She came to a vast room in the middle of this palace, the ceilings. So high she could barely see the top and in the middle was a circular table and on that table was a beautiful ornate clock. She went over to that clock reached out and touched that clock. As she did, the ticking stopped, and as the ticking stopped. So she suddenly realized time may not stand still for any man, but it has stood still for her. Then she touches the hands she slowly with her finger whines. Those hands back, and she doesn't know quite why she feels like this is the thing to do. She rewinds those hands, and as she does, she noticed his life coming back to the castle. This palace sees people appearing almost out of thin air, and then she reaches the point where she's winding. She hears this slight click with the clock, and she feels like that's the place she's supposed to stop winding. So she stops turning moves her finger. Here's the clock chime.

As the clock chimes so all these people start milling around moving. As if life has returned to this palace and someone suddenly startled to see this woman. They didn't know a moment earlier stood at the clock. She knew with this that she'd undone a curse that was brought upon her land that she traveled from that was somehow connected through time and space with this palace. This clock that in her land somehow time ground to halt everyone started disappearing as if they no longer existed. She got out of the area but was aware that this problem was following her not far behind at the rate of one tick per talk. She couldn't explain that, but she knew she was keeping ahead and had a sense that there was a connection between them somehow. She walked through all the people in the palace and went on her journey, able to enjoy. This land more on her journey home, knowing that she had changed her area and helped save the people in her field. Just as much as she had just helped to protect the people in that palace, when she eventually reached back to her area, she was gratefully received. She saw her loved ones saw how happy she'd made everyone. They have had a vague sense that something had happened and that now they were back. She looked forward to just going home after a long journey relaxing down and falling asleep.

Volcano Island

You can have a sense of finding yourself walking through a museum as you walk through that Museum so you can hear the way that your footsteps echo off. The walls you can listen to doors being opened and closing. The way the sounds of the doors echo through the corridor and down into each room and Museum. While you walk around the museum, so you notice that everyone is beginning to leave. But the museum is starting to close for the night. You're here to keep an eye on the paintings the statues when everyone's gone home. So you walk around checking that everyone's leaving the museum. While you walk around, you notice different sculptures, different paintings, large paintings, smaller paintings. You hear the different doors being closed as different rooms are empty of people until eventually, all the customers have left. Then the other staff leave and leave you to keep an eye on the museum yourself. After the last person has left and the front door has been closed, so you go and sit down. Somewhere in one of the rooms and the idea is that you'll sit down in a room. Then every 15 20 minutes, you'll stand up and walk to another room and sit down there for a while.

Just doing the rounds so that you're in each room as the night goes on being still being able to listen in case there are any sounds in the museum. As you sit in one of the rooms, so you hear some sounds. You decide to go and investigate, and what you find in one of the rooms is the sound of tribal drums. Then you can't figure out where that sound is coming from, and then you notice that some of the statues start to come alive. Then one of the icons comes over to you, and you're a little surprised by this. The figure comes over to you and says that your help is needed that you need to find a lost gem, a gem that belongs to one of the figures in the museum. Until that gem is placed back in the figure, things can't settle, and you don't understand exactly why or what they mean, but the way that they describe this makes you think you've got to go and help in some way. You think it's got to be more exciting than just sitting in one room or another in silence.

So you ask what it is you need to do, and the statue looks over at a painting. You walk over to that painting, and as you get to that painting, you gaze into it. You notice how large that art is that the picture is taller than you are and at least twice as wide. You look into that painting, and you can see it's a painting of a volcanic island. A volcanic island containing a forest as you don't know what you're supposed to do, then notice there seems to be something unusual about this painting. There appears to be a slight shimmer to the art, so you reach out with your hand and gently put your fingertips onto the artwork. As you place your fingers onto the painting, your hand starts to go through the canvas, and it feels like your hand is gently lowered into some freshwater. You can contact the surface tension around your fingers. You can think that moving up your fingers to your palm of your hand and then keeping it in your hand.

You can feel it moving to your wrist and then slowly tickling and tingling as it moves up your arm as you push your hair and into the painting. After your arm is in the picture, so you step in and follow it. She finds yourself in that painting on the volcanic island, and you can hear a thunderstorm start to rage here lashes of rain. You begin to get soaking wet see run into the forest and as you run into the woods. You notice how the rain changes you can now hear that rain falling on the leaves above you listen to it bouncing on those leaves here the thwap sound as each large raindrop hits the large leaves. You're relatively dry inside this forest with such dense forest around you, and you can hear the rumble of thunder. Notice shards of light appear from above as the thunder rolls and lightning flashes. You walk through this forest and feel lucky that it's quite warm here as you walk further into the woods.

You start to dry off while being protected from that rain protected from the raging storm. You continue walking further through the forest you don't yet know what you're looking for how you're going to find this gem. Where this gem is and as you continue walking through the forest, so from time to time, you reach out and touch the bark of trees fill that at your fingertips. You can feel the third of each footstep on the ground, the dull thud as the sound gets absorbed by all the woodland you can hear that storm above hear that heavy rain on the leaves. You continue walking more profoundly and more in-depth, and as you keep walking, you don't know where you're going. And there just seems to be a bit more of a path on the route that you're taking. You recall what this picture looked like before you stepped into it. So you try to remember that in your mind, almost like a map trying to work out where you must have appeared. Where you must be now, you know that you're on a volcanic island. You're currently not walking uphill or downhill. You know you're not stepping up towards the center of the island or down directly towards the coast. You must be walking across the island, which means at some point you'll start walking down.

But for now, you're just walking through the forest and after some time of walking through the woods. You start here a bit more wind coming from in front of you, and you realize you must be approaching the edge of the woods. Although most of the rain isn't making its way to you and isn't falling on you, he's being blocked by the canopy above. You're aware that you're going to need to keep dry when you get out the other side. So what you start doing is collecting some of the big leaves around you. You begin collecting some more significant bits of wood, and on some trees, they have bark, which you can cut at the top. Then you can peel it off in strips, almost like a rope. So you do that and get yourself a load of pieces of bark then as you approach the far side of the forest. You start to see some light again, and you know that warm, and yet there's some light because above the storm. The Sun hasn't set yet, and so you clear the forest walking back out into the rain, you see that you're near the edge of a cliff. So you decide to set up a camp here.

You need to set something up that can just keep you dry and protected. You decide you'll continue your search when the storm has passed see make a pyramid with the more significant bits of wood you tie it all into place with bark bits. You weave in the leaves tie some of them into place, creating a watertight shelter. You place some of the other leaves inside, and then you cruel inside your tent and relax down. While you relax down, so the storm rages on, let's light up with lightning, you can hear the rumble of thunder and understand the large raindrops hitting the ground around you hitting your makeshift tent. Now you're in the dry and sitting down; you feel so relaxed. You find the sounds calming relaxing you find their peaceful they make your mind just want to drift and wander, and from where you are, you're looking out off a cliff over the sea. You can see that seas are quite rough at the moment much of its clouded by the falling rain. So while you sit in your makeshift tent, your eyes begin to close. As your eyes start to close, so your mind starts to drift and dream, and you drift and dream and float back through time in your account. You begin to have this sense have almost been like a bad of just flying over the ocean seeing this clear blue sea seeing comfortable rolling waves.

You drift back through time, and you have a sense of wonder about this island. You're on what the island was like before it was an island how did it become this volcanic island, drifting and floating through the time you have this sense of underwater deep down. A volcano is gently erupting lava is spewing out crackling and popping as it reacts with the water glowing red in the deep blue sea as it gradually builds up. This island from deep under the ocean building. This island up higher and higher towards the surface, and you watch in your mind's eye. As that continues at a steady pace and then occasionally, a more massive eruption happens. Under the sea and the island gets a growth spurt, and then after thousands of years, Ireland begins to get nearer to the surface. Then gradually, the whole time, the land over the magma is shifting slightly. The island is gently elongating until, eventually, one day, the tiniest island appeared above the waves. Initially, just creating some ripples on the surface where it was just below the surface most of the time and only at low tide would it be just above the surface.

Until one day, there was this tiny island. Then the volcano continued erupting and grooved 1-meter square island to meet a square island 4-meter square Island 8-meter square Island 16-meter square Island. It started growing exponentially while the whole time, the island was moving. While the magma was remaining in the same place. After a while, there was this vast black island above the surface of the water with nothing. But black rock and then as time continued, so the Earth's plates continued to move. Thus the magma was creating other islands elsewhere and no longer producing this island. Then as thousands of years continue to pass, random seeds are blown. In the breeze around the earth would find themselves caught on the island and then one-day thousands and thousands of years ago the tiniest little sprout of green started growing on the island followed by another and another. Until the island started turning from black to green and then as even more time passed little sprouts of trees began springing up. Suddenly these trees started growing taller and taller and over hundreds of years. They expanded into tall forests encircling the volcanic island.

The water crashed against the island, creating areas of beaches and the other regions of cliffs. Then as thousands of years continued, some life would find its way to the island floating on branches and leaves from other places. The occasionally lost bird landing and making the island their home, and some would survive and find others. Then create more, and others would be the only one of their kind would make the island their home for their life. As thousands and thousands of years passed trees and plants, multiple generations of experience exist on the island. They have lived on the island, then you float around and drift around like a bird. In the sky, they are finding it fascinating looking down on this island, watching the evolution of this island from when it was just forming on the ocean surf on the bottom of the ocean watching. As it grew up to lore until I broke the surface of the ocean became an island that you see now that you recognize as being like the island. You're currently camping on, and your mind drift wanders seas the island.

The most beautiful calm sea with the most beautiful sky as your attention then draws back to the fact you're in a tent. You're in a makeshift shelter on the edge of a cliff gazing out over the ocean with the storm raging around you. And you look out of the tent you see the heavy rain falling in front of you. You hear the sound of the rain on your makeshift shelter. You can see the rough sea and the lighting and darkening of the clouds as lightning rumbles through the sky and as you continue to watch. So you notice how that rumbling thunder how that storm seems to be weakening. You can then see how rain is falling over the ocean and no longer falling over you as you continue watching so as that storm moves further out to sea as that storm passes by towards. The horizon and you watch the way the Lightning dances in the clouds make the tops of the clouds glow and flash and flicker before a low rumbling of thunder reaches your ears. You notice how the sea below you appears to be calming as that storm moves. Further away and after some time you notice the storm has moved far enough away that you can see some glass sky you can see some cloudless sky.

You can notice the red hue to the sky, and you know that somewhere behind that storm, a Sun is setting as you watch that red hue dimming down. You sit there gazing out to sea, watching that storm at night until eventually, the rumbles get so quiet. You can barely make them out, and yet you can still see on her eyes. The way that storms in those clouds high up into the air as lightning dancing flashing and flickering making those clouds glow with white light, almost like a light machine in a party flickering that white light through those clouds. As hours continue to pass, that storm gets more distant until you see that it's almost entirely over the horizon. You can see at the same time the Sun is practically wholly set. There's just the faintest orange glow on the horizon. As the Sunsets over the background and the storm pass by, the sky ends up a cloudless sky, the air smells. So fresh and clean and bright, you can start to hear sounds around you of wildlife. In the forest, so relaxing, then you start gazing up at the sky, gazing up at all the stars seeing more appearing as the light disappears.

And as your eyes begin to get used to the dark and you just gaze up comfortably in awe at the sky feeling—a sense of how small you are when looking at such a blanket of beauty. As you gaze up at that sky, you notice a meteor shower happening. You start to see streaks of light flashing across the sky, in all directions looking like they're coming from a constellation of Leo and you watch as that happens from that constellation. As you watch those meteors flashing across the sky, you feel like you can hear the fizzing and popping. And you know it must be in your mind because you know there's no time for the sound to have reached your ears. Yet because they'd be burning up high in the atmosphere and again, you feel like you can hear the fizzing and popping. You notice some of them are slightly different colors to white;

you even have this sense like you can smell the meteorites. As if they're landing near you almost like the smell of a sparkler. But again, you know that just must be in your mind. Because of how intensely focused you are on the beauty of this, how dark it is be getting here.

While it's getting darker and darker here so you realize you can see the Stars meet yours brighter than you ever could before in your life. You get so drawn into the experience you almost forget that you stepped into a painting. This is all taking place inside an art because you should be in the museum. Yet this all feels so real to you, almost like this is real, it all feels. So real to you, it doesn't feel like you're in a painting, not that you'd know what being in a picture would feel like. So as you continue to gaze up at the sky gaze over the sea, which now looks jet-black, you decide it's time to close your eyes. Rest for the night you'll try and find the gym in the morning so you take a moment to settle down and your makeshift you close your eyes. You fool asleep, and while you sleep, you start to hear the sound of water being pushed aside like always driving through the water. You feel so comfortable that you feel like you're resting and sleeping in that early, dozy state where you can feel asleep.

Yet feel awake at the same time, and you feel so relaxed, and then you start to feel the warmth of the Sun on your face. So you listen to that water around you just the subtle slightest lapping of the water around you the feeling of the warmth of the Sun on you the pushing sound of the water almost like was gently pushing through the water. Then after a few moments, you start to come around, and you begin to open your eyes. You realize you've been sleeping on the back of a giant turtle, and you feel perfectly fine and calm and curious. You start looking around you, and in every direction, all you see is the smoothest most beautiful turquoise e blue water that leads to a turquoise e blue sky. The color of the water and the sky's color are so similar you can't tell the difference between the rain. The air you can't see where the horizon is, you can't know where the sea ends and where the sky begins. You look in front of you, and you look all around you. You look behind you and feel that turtle beneath you the smoothness of its shell as it continues to swim through the ocean.

As it swims so, it could almost be staying stationary because nothing around you changes. You can't see anything you're heading toward or anything you're heading away from you can't see anything to the left or the right of you or anywhere else around you. The perfect blue just surrounds you. After a while, the turtle lowers its head and starts to dive beneath the water's surface. As you dive beneath the water's surface on the turtle's back, you hold on as it falls. You notice straight away that you can breathe underwater just as quickly as you can on the surface. That the turtle is breathing just as soon as it does on the surface. You can hear bubbles of air with each out-breath coming from you coming from the turtle. You can feel the water on you as you push through that water diving deeper and deeper. As you dive deeper, the bottom of the ocean begins to come into view. You can see fish just going about their everyday lives; you can see how seaweed is swaying and moving under the surface of the water. You don't know where you're diving too, or you know as you seem to be diving deeper.

After some time you are diving deeper and deeper, the turtle levels off. It starts to follow what looks almost like a path of pure white sand between two cliffs. It's an extensive path, and after a while, two mermaids appear either side. As if to escort you somewhere and they're swimming along silently either side of the turtle. As you swim on that turtle's back following this path, unsure exactly where you're going, just feeling curious about the experience. Then after you turn a couple of corners so the sides give way to an open plane of whites and whites and that appears to have waves built into it that has rippled across that sand and off. In the distance, you see what looks like a

Crystal Palace. You notice that the turtle is swimming towards that palace and that these mermaids are escorting you towards. This palace and all the fish go about their lives but move out your way as you're heading towards that Palace. Then after a while, you find yourself entering into the palace entrance when you follow along corridor being escorted by these mermaids. At the end of a long corridor is a massive door, and Toomer people open the door stand aside. As the mermaids and the turtle in yourself' pass through into a vast chamber.

The high ceiling chandeliers light glistening and reflecting everywhere merpeople are standing down both sides what looks like a king and queen on Thrones. The turtle lands on the ground, allowing it's headed the mermaids to swim off and join the other people you climb off the turtle's back. You walk your way through the water, finding it easy and effortless to walk through the water, finding it more comfortable than you expected. You walk through the water and stand in front of the king and queen. They tell you that what you seek is rooted in the valley at the end of a cave, and only two legs can find it. You don't know what this means, but you sure this must be something to do with what you're searching for they say to return. After you've got what you seek, so you go back to the turtle climb back onto the turtle shell, the turtle raises its head moves its fins pushing off. The ground is turning around swimming back out of the chamber down the corridor and out of the palace. The turtle swims around the outside of the palace and starts swimming along behind the palace away from the castle.

Further and further until eventually, there appears to be a cliff, and the turtle dive straight down into that cliff going deeper and deeper, under the surface of the ocean, swimming down deeper and further and further and more profound. As the water gets darker and darker, then you notice as you're swimming down deeper. Further, how everything seems to get quieter how it's interesting that time seems to almost standing still underwater, everything seems to be in slow motion. You swim down deeper and deeper, and after some time, you find you can barely see in front. Then you notice that there's some ground approaching, then the turtle follows that ground and swims along and finds the entrance to a cave. You realize you can barely see now there's no way you're going to be able to see in the cave. You start to focus on the solution that you want some light you want to be able to see inside the cave. You start focusing on that solution. You focus on what it is you want as you're focusing on what it is you want. So you find that you can see little green lights starting to flicker all around you, getting closer and brighter and brighter and closer.

You notice a shoal of fish starts to form around you, and the turtle below you above you to leave to the right behind you of bioluminescent fish. They're swimming on the spot or all around you lighting up where you are almost turning the whole of you into a giant torch. Then you think about going into the cave, and the turtle starts into the cave. As the turtle does so, the fish keep pace with you and swims in with you. You notice the green glow of the fish on the walls—the cave on the floor of the cave, the roof of the cave swimming into that cave. You swim more profound and deeper into that cave. I'm sure what you're going to discover is swimming more intelligent and more in-depth.

Further and further, and then you start to notice something in front of you, it looks like off in the distance is a wooden door. You arrive at that wooden door you get off of the turtle you knock on the door and hear the underwater knock you then knock in another location. You try and find a way through the door. You can't find any easy, obvious way, and then you see on the ground two marks that almost looked like footprints.

So you put one foot on one mark one foot on another score, and nothing happens. You bounce around a bit, and still, nothing happens, then you see a mark on the wall on one side and the other side. You reach out, and you put your hands on those marks, and you push in all four directions. At the same time, pushing down with both legs and pushing on the wall with both hands. Then you hear a clunk and notice how that wooden door slides aside. You enter through the wooden door and find yourself inside a large chamber. In the center of that chamber and you notice the way that light seems to be coming from somewhere almost like light is perhaps channeled from the surface. Um, how through the cave-in two beams straight onto that gem, and you see the way that gem is lit up by those beams of light. You pick the gem up off the pedestal notice. It's the most beautiful gem you've ever seen, and you feel that in your fingers. In the palm of your hand, you feel the weight of that you roll it around. Your fingers gently and slowly, and as you do so down into the ground, you can hear the rumble of rock.

As the pedestal lowers and as you notice a little chamber at the back, opening up as a rock door slides aside. She walked the end of the house when he finds a scroll, and you pick up that scroll. Decide to take the scroll and the gem back with you, and you head back you get back on the turtle. You start to swim out of the cave with all those fish surrounding you swim out of the cave. When you get outside the cave, the fish start following you up through the darkness than when you reach a point where the light allows the fish to disperse and swim away. The turtle continues swimming up and then around and heads round to the entrance to the palace. It floats its way into the castle, swims back to the central room lands on the ground. You walk to the king and queen, and you say you found the gem, and they say you can keep the gem. You say you also found the scroll, and they tell you it's a scroll that they've known the existence of but have never been able to get. Yet it's a scroll that can maintain peace across the land, and you hand over the parchment. They thank you for that, and they know that the knowledge the wisdom can be taught to the people of the land taught far and wide to bring peace and comfort.

You walk back to the turtle climb back on the turtle and swim out of the palace swim back out across vast open white flats of sand finding your way. And back to the surface and then when you reach the surface, you notice that nothing has changed. You still can't see anything in any direction. There's still just this beautiful blue, the slightest movement of the water. The sound almost like oars of the turtle swimming through that water. You rest on the back of that turtle as it swims through the water. While it swims through the water, so you rest your cheek on the end of the turtle, you can feel the back of that turtle against your cheek. You can feel the warmth of the Sun. You feel comfort relaxation, and you feel yourself beginning to drift comfortably asleep as you drift comfortably asleep so you can hear in the background the slight sound of the water. The sound of the turtle swimming feels the warmth of the Sun feels your gentle breathing. Gradually the sour begin to fade away; slowly, it all starts to fade away.

You find yourself beginning to hear Siebert beginning to listen to a louder see against the shore in the cliff starting to look. But other sounds in the forest feeling a breeze on your skin. You find yourself back in that tent again in that makeshift tent gazing out off that cliff over the ocean seeing the blue sky, seeing the Sun rising aware that storm has long passed feeling the breeze on your face. You surprised yourself by finding that the gem is in your hand and that somehow that experience on the turtle even though you feel like you fell asleep. It was a dream that was somehow real, but then you're unsure about how real because you're already inside a painting, you fell asleep in art and ends up in the sea on a turtle. You don't question it something feels comfortable about it. So you take that gem you leave your camp, and you head off into the forest, starting to make your way back to where you came from. You walk through the woods, unsure exactly where you're going to go or how you're supposed to get back out of the painting.

You walk through the forest, just trusting yourself walking through our woods, hearing the sounds in the woods the relaxing sounds in the woods the sounds of each footstep. The feeling of breeze the sounds of rustling leaves as the wind blows in the trees finding your way through the woods. Then after a while, you find your way out the other side of the forest, and you see a tree that seems fuzzy. You walk over to that old fuzzy tree you go to touch the bark of that fuzzy tree and find your hand starts going into the tree. So, you put your hand in your arm in, and eventually, you take a step through that tree. You find yourself back in the museum, and you show the living statue of the gem. The statue says that's the gem that was needed the treasure that will help them all to finally sleep and rest that will help everything go back to the way. It should be, and the statue explains why that gem so important and walks you round to a specific statue. In the head of that statue is a gap where this gem should be, then you place that gem in the difference in that statue.

As you do so, the other statue starts walking away back to where it's supposed to be stood. Before it's reached where it's supposed to be held, it grinds to a halt and stops in a standing position, and everything goes silent. You walk back to that painting, and you touch the art, and it's just a typical painting of a volcanic island. You're unsure what to make of your experience as your shift comes to an end. You go home in the morning and pondering. Your knowledge and the meaning of your experience, you go to bed and as you go to bed. So, you fall asleep, and as you fall asleep, so you drift and dream you hear tribal drums. You find yourself on that volcanic island sitting in your makeshift tent, gazing out over the ocean aware that when you fall asleep here in this tent. You'll find yourself awakening on the back of that turtle, awaiting whatever adventures happen next.

CPSIA information can be obtained
at www.ICGtesting.com
Printed in the USA
BVHW041524171120
593515BV00012B/952